The Art, Science, and Strategy of Longevity

AN EXPANSIVE EXPLORATION OF
AGING, HEALTH, AND HUMAN POTENTIAL

The Art, Science, and Strategy of Longevity

AN EXPANSIVE EXPLORATION OF AGING,
HEALTH, AND HUMAN POTENTIAL

Ioulia Howard, MD, and
Don Howard, MD, PhD

Copyright © 2025 by Ioulia Howard and Don Howard
All rights reserved. No part of this publication may be reproduced, stored in a retrieval system, or transmitted in any form or by any means—electronic, mechanical, photocopying, recording, or otherwise—without the prior written permission of the publisher, except in the case of brief quotations used in reviews or scholarly works.

First edition
Published in the United States of America by
Vibrant Ages Publishing
Mercer Island, Washington

ISBNs:
Hardcover: 979-8-9929178-1-9
Paperback: 979-8-9929178-2-6
eBook: 979-8-9929178-0-2

Library of Congress Control Number: 2025906288

For more information, visit: www.vibrantages.com or www.vibrantages.org
For inquiries, contact: time@vibrantages.com

Important Notice to Readers
This book is intended for educational purposes only. It is not a substitute for professional medical advice, diagnosis, or treatment. Always seek the guidance of a qualified healthcare provider with any questions you may have regarding a medical condition, medications, or health-related decisions.

Disclaimer and Limitation of Liability
The information contained in this publication does not constitute medical advice, diagnosis, or treatment. It is solely for informational and educational purposes. The content herein is not a substitute for professional medical judgment or consultation with a qualified healthcare provider. Nothing in this book should be interpreted as an attempt to offer or practice medicine, nor does it establish a physician–patient relationship.

Readers must not use the information in this book to self-diagnose, treat, or manage any health condition or disease. Never disregard, avoid, or delay seeking professional medical advice because of something you have read in this book. All health-related decisions, including those involving the use of medications, supplements, or therapeutic interventions, should be made only in consultation with a licensed medical professional who is familiar with your individual circumstances.

The authors and publisher expressly disclaim all responsibility for any liability, loss, or risk, personal or otherwise, that may be incurred as a direct or indirect consequence of the use and application of any content in this book. Reliance on any information provided in this publication is at the reader's own risk.

"Do not grow old, no matter how long you live. Never cease to stand like curious children before the great mystery into which we were born."
—Albert Einstein

Preface

Aging touches every life, sparking curiosity and uncertainty in equal measure. Long perceived as inevitable decline, growing older now emerges as a dynamic journey influenced by genetics, environment, and deliberate choices. We stand today at a remarkable crossroads, where extraordinary breakthroughs in medicine, biotechnology, and longevity science are dismantling our long-held certainties about aging. Yet, as these advances illuminate new possibilities, they also introduce complexities, underscoring the need for careful guidance in a world where scientific progress often moves faster than public understanding.

Healthy aging extends beyond biological markers—it encompasses emotional, social, and psychological dimensions as well. Throughout our years of clinical experience, we have witnessed firsthand the consequences of neglecting proactive care—physically, emotionally, and socially. Equally, we have encountered remarkable vitality, wisdom, and fulfillment when the process is approached intentionally, emphasizing psychological resilience, robust social ties, and purposeful living.

These clinical insights resonate deeply with our personal experiences. Between us, we've known multiple generations of our families—Ioulia spanning five, Don seven—from great-grandparents to great-grandchildren. These relationships have strengthened our conviction that growing older involves far more than extending lifespan; it means enriching the quality, depth, and meaning of our years. Reflecting on these personal connections, we are reminded of the lighthearted yet insightful quip: *"If I'd known I was going to live this long, I'd have taken better care of myself."* Although its author remains uncertain, this gentle humor underscores a poignant truth—that purposeful aging requires intentional choices made well before they seem necessary.

Aging is neither a script we must follow nor a shadow we must escape. Rather, it is a thought-provoking experience, one we engage with knowingly, influenced day by day through our actions, circumstances, and the knowledge we continually gain. Our collective goal must not simply be to live longer but also to enrich our lives—to preserve clarity, adaptability, and significance, empowering us to actively shape and fully embrace the years ahead.

This book emerged from decades of practice, scientific inquiry, and reflective exploration—experiences closely intertwined with our personal and professional lives. By integrating knowledge from science and medicine with the psychological, emotional, social, and philosophical dimensions of aging, we seek to empower readers as they navigate their individual journeys through life.

We once saw aging as fate. Now, we embrace it as possibility.

Time is not inevitably lost—it is deliberately gained, moment by moment, choice by choice. Through these choices, we craft the story of our lives.

With gratitude and enthusiasm, we invite you to explore and embrace the remarkable journey that lies ahead.

—Drs. Ioulia and Don Howard

Table of Contents

Preface vii

Acknowledgments..xiii

Introduction.. xv

Part I: Understanding Aging—History, Philosophy, and Science.......1

Chapter 1   Aging Across Time: A Historical Perspective 3

Chapter 2   The Art of Aging Well: Philosophical Reflections on Longevity and Meaning..17

Chapter 3   Why We Age: Scientific Theories on Life's Fundamental Mystery...27

Part II: The Foundations of Longevity—Proven Strategies for a Healthier, Longer Life 47

Chapter 4   Movement is Medicine—The Power of Physical Activity 49

Chapter 5   Nutrition for Longevity: The Science Behind Food and Health 65

Chapter 6   Beyond Diet—Supplements and Functional Foods That Work..75

Chapter 7   Fasting and Caloric Restriction: Activating Cellular Renewal..85

Chapter 8	Beyond Rest: Sleep's Secret Role in Longevity and Health	95
Chapter 9	Mental Resilience and Stress Management: Cultivating Inner Strength for Longevity	105
Chapter 10	Emotional and Spiritual Wellness: A Holistic Approach to Aging	111
Chapter 11	The Pleasure Principle: Sexual Intimacy	117
Chapter 12	Mastering the Hormonal Clock: Discovering the Secrets to Aging Gracefully	125
Chapter 13	Hormone Replacement Therapy: Restoring Balance for Optimal Healthspan	135

Part III: Rewriting the Rules of Aging—Longevity Science and Biohacking ... 147

Chapter 14	Rapamycin and Rapalogs: Pioneering the Anti-Aging Frontier	149
Chapter 15	Metformin: Reimagining a Diabetes Drug for Longevity	161
Chapter 16	Boosting NAD+: NMN and NR in Cellular Rejuvenation	171
Chapter 17	Cellular Rejuvenation: Senolytics, Acarbose, and Telomerase in Aging Science	175
Chapter 18	Non-Pharmacological Biohacks: Effective Optimization Without Medication	183

Part IV: Next-Generation Longevity—Personalized Health and Revolutionary Innovation ... 197

| Chapter 19 | Regenerative Medicine: Unlocking Your Body's Healing Potential | 199 |

Chapter 20	Gene Therapy: Editing the Future of Aging	209
Chapter 21	Technology and Longevity: Innovations Shaping Our Healthspan	217
Chapter 22	Artificial Intelligence in Health and Aging: Smarter, Longer Lives	229
Chapter 23	Partnering with Your Healthcare Provider: Building a Longevity Team	241
Chapter 24	From Ambition to Clarity: Crafting Your Personal Longevity Strategy	247

Postscript: The Age of Possibility: A Final Reflection 257

References 259

Acknowledgments

Our deepest gratitude goes to my wife's parents, Alexander and Antonina—both now in their eighties—for their unwavering love, support, and encouragement throughout this journey. Our time spent with them in Russia, especially during the winter months, provided an invaluable opportunity to deeply immerse ourselves in research and concentrate fully on our writing.

Special thanks to Melissa Butterworth, whose thoughtful suggestion initially sparked the idea for this project and guided us onto this rewarding path.

We also wish to acknowledge the valuable support provided by advanced research and reference tools during the preparation, revision, and editorial stages of this book. The insights, perspectives, and conclusions expressed here are entirely our own. We have taken great care to ensure the accuracy and reliability of the information presented; any errors or oversights remain solely our responsibility.

Introduction

*"Aging is an extraordinary process where you become
the person you always should have been."*
—David Bowie

Aging is humanity's oldest enigma—a puzzle that cultures have pondered, scientists have studied, and philosophers have contemplated for millennia. It is both universal and deeply personal, shaping entire societies and individual destinies. Yet aging continues to inspire fascination and provoke fundamental questions about what it means to grow older. Why do we age, and what does aging truly entail? How have our perceptions of aging evolved through the ages, and how can we best respond to this universal human experience now that we stand on the brink of revolutionary breakthroughs?

Historically, societies have grappled with aging in remarkably diverse ways. Some cultures revered their elders as venerable sages, keepers of history and wisdom; others perceived aging primarily as a precursor to decline, isolation, and frailty. Philosophers, from ancient Greece to the Enlightenment, have explored aging's inherent tension between accumulating wisdom and experiencing physical loss, crafting rich traditions of thought around the meaning, value, and inevitability of growing older.

Today, our conversation about aging stands uniquely transformed by groundbreaking scientific advancements. Decades of research have deepened our understanding of the biological mechanisms underpinning aging, offering fresh insights into cellular deterioration, genetic factors, and the complex interplay of environmental influences. Scientists no longer see aging as inevitable wear-and-tear but as a highly intricate, malleable phenomenon—one that, increasingly, we have the power to influence.

This book presents a comprehensive exploration of aging from multiple vantage points, moving beyond survival toward a vision of vibrant living. Beginning with foundational insights into history, philosophy, and biology, it charts a journey through proven strategies for optimizing physical health, cognitive strength, emotional resilience, and spiritual wellness. It also ventures further into exciting frontiers of biohacking, regenerative medicine, and emerging technologies that promise to expand our understanding of aging. Because the many facets of aging and longevity are interconnected, foundational concepts and key scientific principles will surface across chapters, each time enriched by their unique context. This purposeful recurrence highlights the inherent complexity of longevity.

Aging's true significance extends beyond the scientific or historical—it lives in our daily experiences and personal aspirations. This book, therefore, is neither a purely academic exercise nor a clinical handbook. Rather, it serves as a flexible blueprint, guiding readers to consciously craft their own paths—enriched by intention, shaped by informed choices, and attuned to personal values and evolving needs. The stakes are high, the possibilities extraordinary—and the choices we make today ripple outward, shaping not only our futures but those of generations to come.

PART I
Understanding Aging — History, Philosophy, and Science

CHAPTER 1

Aging Across Time: A Historical Perspective

"To know the past is to understand the present."
—Pearl S. Buck

Aging, intricately woven into the fabric of human existence, shapes the narratives societies craft about the passage of time. Throughout history and across cultures, our attitudes toward aging have swung dramatically—oscillating between reverence and dread, celebration and resistance. Some societies honor their elders as treasured living libraries, vessels of wisdom whose insights illuminate pathways for younger generations, preserving collective memory and identity. Others perceive aging predominantly in terms of loss—a gradual fading of strength, beauty, and relevance—sparking an enduring quest to delay, mitigate, or even defy its effects.

These contrasting perspectives have influenced cultural ideals, traditional norms, and medical progress. Civilizations uncomfortable with aging's inevitability have tirelessly sought remedies that promise renewed vitality, from ancient herbal elixirs to today's advanced biotechnology targeting cellular rejuvenation. Amidst this ceaseless pursuit of longevity, a question surfaces: As the frontiers of longevity expand, perhaps our most compelling challenge lies not in lengthening life's narrative, but in deepening the wisdom and wonder within each chapter.

Today, as groundbreaking scientific advances render the once-elusive dream of prolonged youth increasingly attainable, revisiting historical attitudes toward aging gains newfound significance. By reflecting upon how our ancestors grappled with and understood this universal process, we gain invaluable context for contemporary efforts to understand what aging well actually means. Thus, aging emerges not simply as biological destiny, but as an ever-evolving cultural narrative, continually moulded by human imagination, enduring values, and our limitless curiosity about life's possibilities.

The Earliest Views on Aging

In humanity's earliest societies, aging carried an evocative duality—deeply revered for its wisdom, yet shadowed by undeniable fragility. Elders were the foundation upon which their communities stood, valued not only as survivors but as essential keepers of lived experience. They held intimate knowledge of nature's rhythms, anticipating shifting seasons, identifying life-sustaining plants, healing sickness, and sensing hidden dangers long before they emerged. Through shared stories and carefully preserved insights, elders wove threads of continuity, guiding their communities from one generation to the next. Though even as they illuminated the path forward, their growing vulnerability served as an ever-present reminder of life's fleeting beauty and time's steady, relentless progression.

As civilizations flourished, these early reflections on aging deepened and found expression in myths, poetry, and epic narratives. Few stories capture humanity's eternal tension with mortality as poignantly as *The Epic of Gilgamesh*. Within this ancient Mesopotamian masterpiece, Gilgamesh—a figure mighty yet touchingly human—is devastated by the loss of his cherished companion, Enkidu. Grief-stricken and haunted by the certainty of his own mortality, Gilgamesh embarks on a desperate and arduous quest for immortality.

The eternal life he longs for remains just beyond his reach. Instead, Gilgamesh uncovers a truth as timeless as his story: physical immortality is an illusion. True endurance arises not from conquering aging, but from the legacies we cultivate—the wisdom we generously share, the communities we lovingly nurture, and the stories we purposefully pass along. Gilgamesh's transformative journey continues to resonate deeply, reaffirming humanity's oldest wisdom: aging and death are not foes to conquer, but essential currents in the ever-flowing river of human existence.

Gilgamesh's story invites us to reflect on our own lives. As time shapes us, what legacy will we choose to leave behind? How will the years we've been given transcend the limits of our own existence?

Aging in the Ancient World: Wisdom, Decline, and Social Realities

In the ancient world, aging represented a profound duality—revered for its wisdom yet shadowed by inevitable physical decline. Venerated philosophers such as Socrates, Plato, and Aristotle saw advanced age as far more than biological fate; they viewed it as an extraordinary opportunity for intellectual growth and ethical reflection. Aristotle, in particular, considered later life uniquely suited for the cultivation of reason and discernment—faculties polished and sharpened by a lifetime of experience. Even so, he openly acknowledged a bittersweet trade-off: with wisdom's bounty came the certain toll of bodily deterioration.

This philosophical recognition of aging's dual nature—wisdom paired inseparably with decline—was vividly embodied in Greek mythology and symbolism. Central to Greek cultural imagination stood Chronos, the personification of relentless, unstoppable time. His presence was a compelling reminder of human mortality, echoed powerfully through myths and legends. Yet, simultaneously, these same myths expressed humanity's timeless yearning for renewal and immortality—seen in tales of rejuvenating fountains and restorative elixirs. Such stories reveal the ancient conflict between accepting aging's inevitability and the enduring human dream of transcending its boundaries, a tension that remains palpable today in both medical innovation and popular culture.

In ancient Rome, this dynamic played out differently, influenced by class and social privilege. Among the Roman elite, longevity was interpreted as evidence of divine favor or moral achievement—a tangible reward for virtuous living. The distinguished philosopher Cicero eloquently captured this ideal in his seminal work, *De Senectute* (*On Old Age*). To Cicero, aging was not a slow decline into irrelevance but rather an exceptional stage of life, a time for refining character, deepening wisdom, and securing a meaningful legacy. He viewed old age as dignified and enriching—provided one approached it intentionally, with virtue and continued intellectual engagement.

Beneath Rome's philosophical ideals lay harsher realities for those without privilege: the poor, enslaved, and marginalized. Lacking wealth, status, and education, older members of these communities typically endured intensified hardship, vulnerability, and social exclusion. For them, aging was rarely a serene period of philosophical reflection or community reverence; instead, it was marked by frailty, economic uncertainty, and dependence. Their struggles underscored stark inequalities deeply embedded in ancient societies, highlighting how strongly social status shaped individual experiences of growing older.

This enduring tension—aging as both a gateway to wisdom and an inevitable source of decline—continues to resonate in the present. Ancient philosophers illuminated the aspirational dimensions of growing older, even as their societies revealed the harsher truths of aging. Today, this historical perspective challenges us anew, prompting an essential question: How can we ensure dignity, wisdom, and vitality define aging—not only for the privileged few, but for everyone?

Aging in the Medieval World: Wisdom, Faith, and Social Realities

In the medieval world, aging meant far more than a biological certainty—it was intricately interlaced with spiritual beliefs, cultural traditions, and the rhythms of daily life. Across diverse medieval cultures, old age represented not decline, but transformation: a sacred opportunity for introspection, spiritual maturity, and preparation for what lay beyond. Within Hindu and Buddhist traditions, aging signified an intentional shift from worldly attachments toward spiritual awakening. Central to this view was samsara, the eternal cycle of birth, death, and rebirth. Physical decline was not viewed as misfortune but rather as a poignant reminder of life's ephemeral nature, encouraging detachment from material desires. Ascetics, monks, and sages who purposefully withdrew from society in pursuit of deeper truths were revered as guiding lights, embodying wisdom, discipline, and spiritual liberation. Christianity, too, imbued aging with deep spiritual meaning, though in a uniquely distinctive way. For medieval Christians, later years became a sacred stage—a period dedicated to strengthening one's bond with God, reflecting on life's moral choices, and readying the soul for eternity. Biblical figures such as Moses, who guided his people with strength despite advanced years, and Simeon and Anna, the wise elders who recognized the infant Christ as the long-awaited redeemer, exemplify the deep grace, spiritual discernment, and respect attributed to old age. Nevertheless, Christianity stopped short of idealizing aging entirely. Instead, it openly acknowledged physical frailty and suffering as humbling reminders of life's transitory nature. Consequently, bodily decline was reframed as a sacred journey, purifying and readying the soul for eternal redemption.

Aging was understood through more than just the cultural filter of religion; it was also experienced amid complex social realities. Elders occupied indispensable roles as guardians of collective wisdom, maintaining stability, transmitting knowledge, and safeguarding traditions. Especially in rural communities where formal education was rare, older adults offered essential mentorship—teaching younger generations crucial skills for survival, farming, healing, and preserving history through oral traditions. Their steady presence provided continuity and reassurance in times marked by war, famine, and upheaval. Despite these respected roles, longevity remained exceptional—and consequently, somewhat precarious.

Medieval life, often harsh and uncertain, was marked by disease, violence, and scarcity, resulting in relatively short lifespans. Those who reached advanced age thus occupied an ambiguous position within society. Longevity might reflect divine favor, moral virtue, or exceptional resilience, inspiring admiration and reverence. However, particularly during societal crises, older adults—often women—could provoke suspicion, distrust, or even accusations of witchcraft. Their very existence challenged prevailing norms, revealing deep-seated anxieties surrounding aging's enigmatic nature. This inherent duality—aging as both revered wisdom and troubling vulnerability—captures the complexity of medieval perspectives. Aging during this era was neither purely biological nor exclusively spiritual; rather, it unfolded at the crossroads of religion, culture, economics, and personal circumstance. Reflecting upon these historical insights deepens our contemporary understanding, reminding us that modern attitudes toward aging remain intricately shaped by centuries of evolving beliefs and social conditions. Thus, exploring the medieval experience of aging reveals not a narrative of spiritual insight or physical decline, but a layered portrait of elders navigating reverence, uncertainty, and adversity. Their lives, etched by resilience and adaptability, illuminate the timeless human capacity to create meaning even amid intense hardship and uncertainty.

The Renaissance and Enlightenment: Aging in a New Light

The Renaissance transformed society's view of aging, inspired by a renewed fascination with humanism and the complexities of lived experience. Across Europe, as art blossomed, science advanced, and philosophy deepened, aging emerged prominently as a subject of artistic admiration and intellectual reflection. Master artists, notably Leonardo da Vinci and Michelangelo, captured the aging body with exquisite sensitivity—faces etched by wisdom, hands dignified by labor, forms softened by years. Rather than depicting decline, their work celebrated aging as resilience, dignity, and depth. In elevating old age from biological inevitability to aesthetic reverence, these visionaries endowed it with timeless philosophical significance.

This artistic awakening ran parallel to groundbreaking scientific inquiry, marking a pivotal shift in understanding human aging. The body, once considered a sacred and immutable mystery, became an object of careful, systematic investigation. Anatomists such as Andreas Vesalius ventured into previously uncharted territories through detailed dissections, laying the foundations of modern physiology. While their grasp of aging's intricate biology remained limited, their work signified a critical conceptual shift: aging was no longer fate—it had become a phenomenon open to exploration, observation, and perhaps even intervention.

The Enlightenment deepened and broadened this intellectual transformation, championing reason, human potential, and lifelong intellectual growth. Philosophers like Voltaire and Rousseau challenged prevailing views that equated aging with decline. Instead, they reframed later life as uniquely suited for reflection, intellectual discovery, and personal growth. Rousseau envisioned old age as liberating—a phase where one could step away from the distractions of youth to contemplate deeper philosophical truths. Similarly, Voltaire wisely remarked, "The longer we dwell on our misfortunes, the greater is their power to harm us," suggesting that aging, approached thoughtfully, could become a time of genuine personal fulfillment. Enlightenment ideals thus nurtured a powerful belief: intellectual vitality could not only persist but flourish well into the later chapters of life.

Underlying this optimism lay emerging cultural tensions, tensions that continue to shape contemporary attitudes. Even as elders retained their respected status as guardians of wisdom, Enlightenment values emphasizing innovation and relentless progress began to associate vigor and productivity more closely with youth. The rise of industrialization further intensified this shift, prioritizing attributes such as physical strength, adaptability, and efficiency—qualities often attributed primarily to the young. Gradually, older adults came to be viewed not just as repositories of valuable historical memory and life experience but also as symbols of stagnation, inefficiency, and obsolescence. Thus, industrialization quietly planted the seeds of modern ageism, establishing a cultural bias favoring youth that persists even now.

The Renaissance and Enlightenment stand as transformative eras in humanity's ongoing dialogue about aging. Old age was simultaneously celebrated for wisdom and potential intellectual fulfillment, yet increasingly scrutinized as a hindrance to innovation and progress. This duality, deeply embedded within contemporary society, continually challenges us to reconcile reverence for age-earned wisdom with the societal idealization of youthfulness. How we navigate this tension—whether by reinforcing unspoken ageist biases or embracing aging as an enriched, meaningful stage of life—remains a complex yet crucial question. It is a conversation that began long ago, shaped by the voices of artists, philosophers, and scientists whose insights still resonate today.

The Industrial Revolution: Aging in a Changing World

The Industrial Revolution transformed society, reshaping the meaning and experience of aging. As agrarian lifestyles yielded to industrial economies, traditional family structures—once the cornerstone of elder care and support—began to unravel. Historically, rural elders had served as custodians of cultural wisdom, mentors guiding younger generations, and stabilizing forces within their communities. Yet as younger family members flocked to rapidly expanding cities in pursuit of employment, many older adults found themselves left behind, their roles diminished and their societal value eroded. Even those elders who followed faced unanticipated struggles, navigating urban landscapes devoid of the familiar intergenerational bonds that had long sustained them. In this new social reality, the fabric that had safeguarded older generations began to fray, leaving many increasingly vulnerable to isolation and neglect.

At the heart of industrialization was an uncompromising drive toward efficiency, productivity, and relentless economic growth. Within this shifting landscape, aging—inevitably accompanied by gradual physical and cognitive changes—began losing its traditional association with wisdom and respected experience. Older workers, struggling to keep pace with the harsh demands of factory labor, often found themselves marginalized and perceived as inefficient or expendable. This shift was more than an economic adjustment; it marked a cultural transformation, recasting aging from a respected, natural stage of life into an apparent obstacle to progress. Here were planted the seeds of modern ageism, biases favoring youth and productivity that continue to echo through our societal perceptions today.

The legacy of the Industrial Revolution was not only one of marginalization. The same era that disrupted traditional support networks also ignited an unprecedented exploration of aging. The nineteenth century brought extraordinary advances in medical knowledge and saw the emergence of gerontology as a systematic field of study. Researchers moved beyond philosophical speculation, diving deeper into concrete biological processes—cellular degeneration, declining organ functions, and factors influencing longevity. These pioneering studies aimed not only to extend lifespan but to enhance quality of life, laying essential foundations for modern longevity science. Concurrently, widespread public health initiatives dramatically reduced infectious diseases that disproportionately impacted older populations, fundamentally altering the lived experience of aging.

The Industrial Revolution left behind a complex, dual legacy. On one hand, it dismantled established intergenerational bonds, framing aging as a hindrance to economic efficiency. On the other, it spurred groundbreaking scientific progress, reframing the concept of aging from inevitable decline to a dynamic, potentially modifiable phenomenon. This dialectic—between marginalization and innovation—still shapes contemporary discourse around aging. Today, society remains poised between reverence for elder wisdom and deeply entrenched biases favoring youthfulness. This nuanced debate, with its distinctly modern challenges, can trace its roots directly to the transformative upheavals of the Industrial Revolution.

The 20th Century: Aging as a Scientific Frontier

In the 20th century, aging evolved from life's inevitable conclusion into an expansive landscape of scientific discovery and potential. Breakthroughs in medicine and public health—antibiotics, vaccines, improved sanitation, and better nutrition—sparked unprecedented gains in human lifespan. Aging ceased to be viewed as a fixed biological destiny and instead emerged as a promising realm ripe for systematic investigation, deeper understanding, and perhaps transformative intervention.

Scientists began unraveling the cellular mysteries of aging, identifying processes such as oxidative stress—the damage inflicted by unstable, oxygen-rich molecules—as well as DNA deterioration and telomere shortening, the gradual erosion of protective chromosome end-caps. Genetic research further illuminated these complexities, revealing longevity-associated genes like FOXO, which bolster cellular resilience, and metabolic pathways such as mTOR, a critical regulator of cell growth and metabolism. For the first time in history, a provocative question took center stage: could aging be slowed or even reversed? From this daring inquiry arose the dynamic field of biogerontology, committed not just to extending lifespan, but to enriching healthspan—the years spent unburdened by chronic disease or disability.

Even as science expanded the boundaries of longevity, societal perceptions of aging grew increasingly complex—and often contradictory. Older adults were celebrated for their extraordinary contributions to history, politics, and culture, exemplified by towering figures such as Winston Churchill, Eleanor Roosevelt, and Pablo Picasso. These individuals embodied the inspiring idea that creativity, leadership, and influence could flourish well beyond youth, challenging traditional notions of age-related decline. Simultaneously, however, cultural trends fueled by media increasingly idealized youth, positioning it as the ultimate standard of beauty, vitality, and productivity. Industries like fashion, advertising, and entertainment reinforced these ageist stereotypes, marginalizing older adults, particularly in workplaces where seasoned experience frequently yielded to preferences for youthful vigor.

As global populations grew older, societal structures evolved in response, prompting new policies and support systems designed for an aging world. Initiatives such as the establishment of Social Security in the United States, the rise of retirement communities, and the proliferation of senior-care facilities sought to provide financial security, accessible healthcare, and social engagement. Yet, these developments also laid bare persistent social tensions, prompting debates about dignity, autonomy, and equity—issues that resonate deeply in contemporary conversations about aging.

The 20th century's legacy is a paradoxical blend of scientific triumph and cultural ambivalence. Medical advancements ignited optimism that both life and vitality could be prolonged, even as shifting societal values exposed contradictions—simultaneously honoring the wisdom of older adults while idolizing youth. This transformative era posited aging as an intricate intersection of scientific discovery and cultural dialogue, compelling contemporary society to grapple with the ethical, social, and medical complexities embedded in longevity.

The 21st Century: The Transformation of Aging

Today, aging inhabits a remarkable moment of evolution, defined by extraordinary leaps in science, technology, and shifting cultural perceptions. Once considered life's inescapable script, aging has become humanity's most intriguing narrative—dynamic, adaptable, and open to revision.

Scientific advances have illuminated the complex molecular dance underlying the aging process, revealing intricate mechanisms such as cellular senescence, mitochondrial dysfunction, and epigenetic drift. These insights have ignited a revolution in longevity science, leading fields like geroscience and regenerative medicine to target the fundamental biology of aging. Breakthrough technologies—from precision gene editing (CRISPR) and AI-driven diagnostics to stem cell therapies and senolytic drugs—promise more than extending lifespan. They offer the chance to preserve vitality, cognitive sharpness, and robust health well into advanced age. These groundbreaking innovations and the science behind them will be explored comprehensively in the chapters ahead.

Parallel to these medical innovations, society's perception of later life is undergoing a transformation. Contemporary culture increasingly celebrates older adulthood as a flourishing chapter of continued creativity, reinvention, and meaningful contribution. Movements emphasizing "successful aging" encourage older adults to defy traditional stereotypes—launching entrepreneurial ventures, crafting powerful art, and setting new athletic milestones. In doing so, they reimagine potential, challenging conventional expectations of what life's later stages can hold.

Even amid these promising shifts, ageist biases linger stubbornly. Experienced professionals still encounter discrimination in workplaces that prioritize youth over wisdom. Media and entertainment frequently perpetuate simplistic portrayals of older adults, reinforcing perceptions of diminished capability and relevance. Within healthcare settings, assumptions about inevitable frailty often limit proactive care and prevent opportunities for improved quality of life. Such biases erode individual dignity and rob society of the insights, skills, and talents older generations have to offer.

Beyond these challenges, however, the 21st century has also ushered in greater recognition of the emotional and social dimensions of aging. Concepts like lifelong learning and intergenerational collaboration are dissolving artificial divides between age groups, nurturing mutual respect, empathy, and collective growth. Globally, communities are embracing age-inclusive initiatives—accessible housing, innovative smart-home technologies, supportive social programs, and intentionally designed public spaces—that empower older adults, preserving their independence, fostering engagement, and strengthening social connections.

The experience of growing older today occupies an exciting intersection of groundbreaking scientific discovery and transformative cultural shifts, blending traditional perspectives with innovative possibilities. Far from passive resignation, later life has evolved into an intentional, purposeful stage, guided by informed personal choices and supported by collective strategies. Viewed historically, aging in the 21st century marks a pivotal intersection—where humanity's enduring struggle with mortality meets paradigm-shifting scientific and cultural advancements, reframing both the experience and deeper meaning of longevity.

The Next Chapter: Reimagining Aging for the Future

The process of growing older has always been inextricably linked with the human story—shaping cultures, traditions, and identities across countless generations. From ancient societies that honored elders as guardians of wisdom, to modern pursuits aimed at extending the human lifespan, our relationship with aging has continually shifted between reverence and resistance. Throughout history, we have embraced growing older as part of nature's cycle, confronted it as an obstacle to overcome, and pondered it as one of life's enduring mysteries.

Today, advances in biotechnology, medicine, and longevity science are unveiling groundbreaking discoveries that reconceptualize what it means to age—not as inevitable decline, but as a dynamic biological journey we can study, influence, and perhaps even transform. Alongside the exhilarating promise of extended years emerges a deeper, more challenging question: How do we ensure those years are defined not by survival alone, but by meaningful engagement, genuine autonomy, and a sense of purpose? In the end, longevity itself is not the ultimate measure. What truly matters is the depth, intention, and significance with which we embrace the time we have.

This shared journey extends beyond the physical realm—it shapes our identities, relationships, and the legacies we leave behind. It influences how we perceive ourselves and how we connect with others, guiding the impressions we make and the stories we tell. At its core, the passage through life tests our resilience and invites spiritual adaptability, offering unique moments of introspection, renewal, and rediscovery. In the end, it prompts deep reflection: What does it mean to live with significance—not only in the vigor of youth, but throughout every stage of life?

As science deepens our understanding of aging, we increasingly appreciate that this universal journey reveals far more than biology—it illuminates our collective human narrative. History shows us how societies across time have grappled with the meaning of growing older, each generation adding new layers of interpretation and understanding. Aging becomes a story of continuity and reinvention, shaped by cultural values, societal structures, and evolving perceptions of life's meaning. Looking forward, the future of longevity calls upon these historical insights, urging us not only to extend life, but to enrich it—honoring lessons from the past, savoring the opportunities of the present, and approaching tomorrow with curiosity, wisdom, and a renewed sense of direction.

CHAPTER 2

The Art of Aging Well: Philosophical Reflections on Longevity and Meaning

"The mind is its own place, and in itself can make a heaven of hell, a hell of heaven."
—JOHN MILTON, PARADISE LOST

Aging is more than a biological phenomenon; it is a uniquely human experience that unfolds across time and memory. It echoes through the corridors of our existence—profound, poignant, and endlessly thought-provoking—prompting us to consider some of the deepest mysteries of the universe: the fluidity of identity, the pursuit of purpose, and the inevitability of mortality. As science tirelessly strives to prolong life and safeguard health, philosophy urges a deeper contemplation: What does it mean to live well and fully throughout all our years?

Throughout centuries, great thinkers have grappled with this perennial inquiry, painting aging either as an enlightening pathway toward wisdom or as a gradual descent into decline. Some have envisioned growing older as a portal to richer understanding, a season when life's accumulated experiences distill clarity and strengthen character. Others, however, have depicted it as a quiet unraveling, an erosion of youthful vigor and social significance. How can such sharply contrasting perceptions coexist? What does this duality reveal about our ongoing effort to frame aging?

Philosophical thought has deeply influenced cultural attitudes toward aging, offering lessons about resilience, acceptance, and humanity's quest for purpose amidst change. Across diverse traditions, philosophy offers guidance not only in navigating life's later chapters but in embracing their transformative potential. Even amidst today's unprecedented medical and technological breakthroughs, these ancient teachings remain strikingly relevant, reminding us that longevity does not guarantee satisfaction or happiness.

If granted additional time, how would we spend it most meaningfully? What defines an existence not only lived but richly experienced? This chapter invites readers to explore philosophical traditions—drawing upon ancient wisdom and contemporary perspectives—to reimagine aging. Through these perspectives, aging emerges not only as a challenge to overcome but as an essential space for reflection, offering continual opportunities to clarify life's purpose and deepen our understanding of self.

Ancient Perceptions: How the Great Thinkers Saw Aging

The experience of growing older traces its arc through every human life, not as decline, but as a reckoning with time, identity, and the shifting contours of the self. Long before science sought ways to delay or reverse aging, philosophers grappled with its implications. Across cultures and centuries, a common understanding emerges: the later stages of life are not the gradual erosion of time but constitute a chapter rich with possibility, reflection, and transformation.

The Stoics approached aging with calm acceptance, viewing it with the same clarity and composure they brought to all of life's uncertainties. They recognized that advancing years are inevitable—utterly beyond our control—and thus unworthy of lament. Resisting this natural process, they believed, meant waging a futile battle against nature, inevitably leading only to frustration. Instead, welcoming maturity with grace fostered resilience, wisdom, and inner peace. Central to this outlook was the Stoic ideal of *amor fati*, or "love of fate," encouraging a wholehearted acceptance of life's later chapters rather than fear or avoidance.

Marcus Aurelius, reflecting in his *Meditations*, reminded himself daily of life's fleeting nature. By cultivating virtue and integrity rather than desperately clinging to youth, he sought to approach old age not with regret but with strength. Seneca went further still, boldly asserting that life is measured not by length but by depth—a timeless reminder that resonates perhaps more powerfully today than ever. For the Stoics, virtue—the highest good—meant living harmoniously with reason and nature, with the passage of years integral to this harmony.

Where the Stoics saw life's progression as a test of resilience and virtue, Aristotle viewed it as life's culminating chapter—a fulfillment rather than a loss. His philosophy of *eudaimonia*, often translated as human flourishing, suggested that genuine meaning arises not from fleeting pleasures nor youthful strength but from purposeful, reflective, and virtuous living. Aristotle understood virtue not as moral correctness but as a lifelong commitment to intellectual growth, ethical refinement, and thoughtful moderation. His Doctrine of the Mean emphasized balance: the careful path between excess and deficiency. Older adulthood, he believed, provides the ideal setting to achieve this equilibrium, tempering youthful impulsivity with seasoned insight.

Rather than a period of deterioration, Aristotle celebrated the later years as a stage when wisdom and character reach their fullest bloom. The twilight of life, he argued, offers space for deeper contemplation, richer relationships, and the fine-tuning of ethical pursuits. In striking contrast to modern culture's fixation on youth as the pinnacle of worth, Aristotle acknowledged the quiet grace that comes with experience—a subtler, more nuanced understanding of life's complexities.

While Aristotle highlighted intellectual cultivation, Eastern traditions introduced another dimension: harmony with nature rather than mastery over it. Taoism, through Laozi's teachings, portrays the process of growing older not as a problem needing solutions but as a natural unfolding to approach with ease. Central to this approach is *wu wei*—effortless action—encouraging alignment with life's flow rather than resistance. Like water gliding effortlessly around stones in a stream, Taoism suggests maturing gracefully means adapting smoothly and naturally, without conflict or force.

Buddhism, too, presents a vision rooted in acceptance. The principle of *anicca*, or impermanence, underscores the transient nature of all things. Clinging tightly to youth, vitality, or identity only magnifies suffering. Unlike Stoicism's disciplined acceptance, Buddhism views letting go as liberation—freedom from the pain of attachment. Buddhist teachings foster detachment, discernment, and serenity, reframing older age not as loss, but as an opening for compassion, understanding, and inner peace. Zen practitioners, through seated meditation (*zazen*), train the mind to release past regrets and future anxieties, fully inhabiting the present moment with calm clarity.

While Western traditions often emphasize autonomy, Confucian philosophy regards elderhood as a transition into respected leadership. Elders become guides and mentors, responsible for nurturing younger generations' moral and intellectual development. Central to this is *xiao*, filial piety, an ethical principle underscoring respect for elders as repositories of invaluable knowledge. Unlike modern individualistic societies, where advancing age is sometimes equated with diminishing relevance, Confucian culture cherishes older generations as living links between past traditions and future growth.

Zen Buddhism, however, offers yet another shade of understanding—a more introspective exploration of life's later chapters. Rather than focusing on societal roles, Zen invites an intimate awareness of one's relationship with time. Its teachings promote radical presence, illuminating how suffering arises from attachments to the past or anxieties about the future. Zen philosophy encourages accepting each moment exactly as it unfolds, allowing the natural progression of life to occur effortlessly. Mindfulness and meditation thus illuminate the later years not as something feared but as an open invitation toward clarity, acceptance, and equanimity.

These ancient perspectives challenge today's pervasive fear of growing older, offering timeless lessons about resilience, fulfillment, and serenity. They encourage us to reconsider this stage of life not as deterioration but as continuing evolution—an ongoing process of growth, adaptation, and refinement. Taken together, these philosophies portray aging not as a slow retreat from life but as an artful collaboration with time—encouraging us to harmonize gracefully with change and draw meaning from the wisdom of experience.

The Modern Age: Aging in an Era of Scientific Progress

For most of human history, aging was an unyielding reality—fixed firmly by fate, fortune, and nature's immutable order. Today, that certainty has fractured. Advances once relegated to the realm of science fiction now reshape the trajectory of human aging. Regenerative therapies mend tissues once thought irreparable; precise gene-editing tools recalibrate the cellular clock; pharmaceuticals dismantle senescent cells; and molecular interventions amplify our bodies' innate repair mechanisms. The promise is striking—not just prolonged life, but extended vitality, richer health, and greater well-being.

Amid this astonishing progress, an unsettling question remains: If aging is no longer simply a gradual descent into decline, how can we ensure these extra years are worthwhile?

This dilemma defines modern aging. Society venerates youth—equating it with ambition, vitality, and productivity—while often relegating older adults to the margins. Popular culture echoes this bias: youthful beauty is idolized, dynamic lifestyles glorified, and professional achievement prized above all else. Meanwhile, older people often confront workplace discrimination, social invisibility, and narratives framing aging as withdrawal rather than transformation. As longevity stretches further ahead, a greater challenge, a greater question emerges—what does it mean to age with intention.

Science, for all its wonders, can extend life, but it cannot instruct us on how best to live it. Here, philosophy steps into the silence, offering pathways toward wisdom and understanding. Existentialist thought, especially, has long confronted the question of living well in the face of life's fleeting nature. Unlike traditional thought that grounded life's purpose in external values—the Stoics' virtue, Aristotle's *eudaimonia*, or religious paths toward enlightenment—existentialism argues that meaning is never simply received; it must be actively and deliberately created.

Viktor Frankl, in *Man's Search for Meaning*, asserted that even in the darkest moments, we retain the capacity—and the responsibility—to choose meaning. Frankl, shaped by his experiences as a Holocaust survivor, did not see purpose as something fate hands us, but as something courageously constructed. In this light, aging becomes not loss, but an opportunity—an invitation toward deeper, deliberate living.

Jean-Paul Sartre took this idea further, famously declaring, "existence precedes essence." Human beings, Sartre insisted, arrive without predetermined identities or destinies; instead, each must actively shape their own purpose through thoughtful choice and authentic action. Rather than yielding to decline, aging thus becomes an ongoing process of self-definition—a continual act of reinvention and conscious engagement with existence.

Martin Heidegger expanded existential thought further still, emphasizing the crucial importance of confronting our mortality. Too often, he observed, we drift aimlessly—trapped in routines shaped by societal expectations rather than genuine aspirations, a disengagement that deepens as we age. Heidegger offered a powerful insight: fully acknowledging life's finite nature inspires us toward greater presence, clarity, and deliberate living. Aging, then, is not the passage of time but a summons toward authenticity—a call to focus on what matters most.

Modern society grants remarkable longevity—but longevity does not guarantee fulfillment. Intentional aging requires more than scientific innovation; it calls for a thoughtful philosophy that embraces rather than resists the passage of time, seeing later life not as a conclusion but a continued exploration of potential. Perhaps this involves shifting focus from outward achievements toward inner satisfaction—deepening relationships, nurturing creativity, exploring lifelong passions, or mentoring younger generations. Whatever path is chosen, meaningful aging demands mindful and active participation in the world around us.

Ultimately, today's unprecedented scientific advances compel society to confront a fundamental practical and ethical challenge: building a culture that values extended lifespans, ensuring aging remains a dignified, inclusive, and socially rewarding experience.

The Art of Aging: Philosophical Insights on Longevity and Identity

Contemporary philosophy provides essential perspectives on aging and longevity, exploring the ethical, social, and existential implications arising from rapid advancements in medical technology. As scientific breakthroughs increasingly prolong human lifespan, philosophical inquiry encourages further reflection on the impact these developments hold for humanity. In modern culture, aging frequently carries negative connotations—as something to resist, delay, or reverse—a narrative perpetuated by industries emphasizing perpetual youth. Philosophers challenge this narrow perspective, redefining aging as a valuable stage of life filled with opportunities for personal growth, rewarding relationships, and reflective self-discovery.

Two compelling modern philosophical perspectives merit thoughtful examination of the complex issues surrounding aging. The first, Biotechnological Optimism—often identified as Transhumanism—embraces the frontier of scientific advancement. Advocates highlight genetic therapies, regenerative medicine, personalized healthcare, and artificial intelligence, viewing these innovations as transformative for human life. They envision progress enriching our experiences, enhancing capacities, and expanding possibilities for healthy living. Think of older adults empowered with renewed autonomy. Independence becomes not fleeting, but a lasting reality, supported by technology tailored precisely to individual needs. Yet this hopeful vision requires ethical vigilance. Advocates stress our collective responsibility to distribute these remarkable benefits equitably, guided by fairness, dignity, and social justice. Technological gifts must uplift humanity collectively—not privilege only a fortunate few.

In contrast, Bioconservatism—or Existential Caution—offers an introspective counterpoint. Proponents encourage contemplation of aging's deeper significance. Life's finitude, they argue, lends meaning, authenticity, and immediacy to our experiences. Awareness of mortality inspires us to cherish relationships, prioritize fulfilling pursuits, and savor life's moments with intensity. However, supporters caution against aggressive efforts to extend lifespan through technological means. Such interventions risk straining familial bonds and societal cohesion. Pushing against natural boundaries could unintentionally pressure shared environmental and economic resources. In the end, they assert, this might erode the intrinsic value and rich depth derived precisely from life's inherent boundaries. This perspective suggests that aging involves navigating life's rhythms with grace rather than attempting to override them entirely.

Both philosophical approaches extend their implications into everyday realities like caregiving and dependency. Philosophers reconceptualizing caregiving suggest that dependency is neither vulnerability to be solved by technology nor a natural limitation to be accepted passively. Instead, caregiving emerges as a dynamic expression of human interdependence, enriched by dignity, empathy, and mutual respect. Such an integrated perspective underscores the value of combining technological advancements with ethical sensitivity, enriching human experiences rather than just extending lifespan.

Aging with Intention: Philosophy as a Practical Guide

Philosophy invites us beneath life's surface, uncovering deeper significance within the natural rhythms of aging. Drawing from this wisdom, we understand aging as more than the passage of years—rather, it unfolds as a journey toward authenticity and purposeful living. Stoic acceptance, Aristotelian flourishing, Taoist harmony, and existential courage each provide distinct perspectives. Aging thus emerges not as a curse but as a path toward self-understanding.

Practically applying these philosophical principles enriches daily life. Older adults need not passively accept limiting narratives. Instead, pursuing activities that align closely with personal interests and capabilities makes aging vibrant and rewarding. Regular physical activity suited to individual abilities, mindful nutritional choices, intellectual exploration, and creative pursuits like art, music, or writing transform aging into an inspiring life chapter.

Communities and policymakers play critical roles by fostering supportive environments. Strategic initiatives—such as universally accessible spaces, adaptive housing, intuitive technologies, and intergenerational mentorship—promote independence and dignity. Philosophical reflection also inspires advocacy for inclusive healthcare systems, equitable access to longevity treatments, culturally responsive healthcare services, and targeted outreach, ensuring respect and justice in later life.

Compassionate caregiving anchors these ideals, emphasizing autonomy, respect, and mutual understanding. Programs like respite care, caregiver education, and robust community networks offer essential support, allowing aging to become a time of creativity and meaningful contribution, genuinely valued by society.

Aging well involves crafting a life deeply engaged with others and aligned with personal values and aspirations. Philosophy empowers this process, transforming aging from something endured into an affirmation of our shared humanity—a testament to growth, resilience, and active engagement.

Aging well is both art and philosophy—an integration of reflective wisdom and deliberate choices. Beyond passing years, aging represents an exploration of identity, purpose, and connection. Ancient philosophical traditions offer timeless guidance toward acceptance and insight, while contemporary thought reframes aging as an intentional journey toward continued growth. Standing at the crossroads of age-old wisdom and modern insight, aging reveals itself as a richly rewarding journey toward heightened self-awareness, deeper relationships, and fulfilling experiences—inviting us to reflect on what constitutes true success, celebrate our connections, and embrace each moment.

CHAPTER 3

Why We Age: Scientific Theories on Life's Fundamental Mystery

"Youth is a perpetual intoxication; it is a fever of the mind. Aging is what leads us toward maturity, reflection, and deeper wisdom—it is life's own narrative of discovery."
—MILAN KUNDERA

Aging touches every living thing, yet it remains one of nature's most intricate and fascinating processes. All organisms age. It is a universal story, visible through physical transformations, persistent physiological decline, and an ever-growing vulnerability to illness. For centuries, scientists have grappled with a deceptively simple yet profound question: Why do we age? In seeking answers, numerous theories have emerged—each illuminating distinct facets of a beautifully complex interplay among biology, genetics, and environment.

Yet no single theory fully captures the essence of aging. Instead, these ideas interlace, reinforcing one another, forming a richly textured narrative. Together, they shape our modern understanding of longevity, aging, and the delicate dance between health and decline.

This chapter explores the most influential theories, examining their underlying mechanisms and highlighting their interconnected contributions. By tracing these scientific pathways. we deepen our appreciation of aging—not simply as an inevitability, but as an intriguing, multi-layered journey. Aging, when embraced as a dynamic choreography of biology and experience, transforms from something to dread into an extraordinary narrative—rich with opportunities for insight, meaning, and personal evolution.

The Damage Accumulation Theory: Aging as Biological Erosion

Picture an intricate, carefully maintained clockwork—a complex mechanism humming reliably for years. Gradually, tiny imperfections accumulate; gears lose their alignment, springs slowly weaken, and the system's precision inevitably begins to falter. Aging, according to the Damage Accumulation Theory, mirrors this slow erosion of function. Over time, cellular and molecular damage steadily accumulates, gradually undermining our body's remarkable capacity for self-repair and renewal. Both internal metabolic processes and external environmental stressors act as relentless forces, incrementally accelerating biological decline along converging pathways.

Central to this process of deterioration are mitochondria, the cellular structures often celebrated as the body's microscopic power plants. These tiny organelles tirelessly produce energy essential for life, but there's a cost: energy production generates reactive oxygen species (ROS), unstable molecules akin to stray sparks escaping from a fire. Normally, the body's antioxidant defenses swiftly neutralize these sparks, maintaining a delicate equilibrium. However, with advancing age, these defenses gradually lose their vigor, allowing oxidative stress—the imbalance favoring ROS—to progressively damage DNA, proteins, and cellular membranes. This cumulative oxidative injury erodes cellular integrity, impairing function at the microscopic level and ultimately manifesting as the visible markers of aging.

But internal processes are not solely responsible. External environmental forces intensify this biological erosion. Consider ultraviolet (UV) radiation, encountered daily with every sunny stroll outdoors. UV rays continually bombard skin cells, triggering persistent genetic disruptions—such as pyrimidine dimers, which distort DNA structure and impair cellular repair mechanisms. Similarly, airborne pollutants, including fine particulate matter (PM2.5), invade our respiratory systems, triggering chronic inflammation. Imagine the lungs as embattled landscapes, persistently under siege by microscopic irritants that heighten susceptibility to heart disease and respiratory conditions.

Lifestyle choices further accelerate these cumulative damages. Take smoking, for instance: every inhalation floods cells with toxins, dramatically magnifying oxidative damage and hastening molecular deterioration. Internally, proteins may occasionally misfold, forming tangled clusters within cells. Not every misfolded protein causes disease, but substantial aggregations, such as the amyloid plaques characteristic of Alzheimer's disease or the neurofibrillary tangles seen in Parkinson's disease, significantly increase risk, highlighting the peril of unchecked molecular accumulation.

Aging isn't only physical. Emotional experiences—once considered intangible and separate from biology—are now recognized as powerful accelerators of aging itself. Chronic psychological stress activates the hypothalamic-pituitary-adrenal (HPA) axis, flooding the bloodstream with cortisol, a stress hormone that provokes widespread inflammation and cellular wear. Picture someone burdened by prolonged caregiving, financial insecurity, or loneliness, their cells continually bathed in stress-induced biochemical signals. Over months and years, this persistent stress accelerates biological aging markers, such as telomere shortening—the gradual erosion of protective DNA caps—exposing cells to further vulnerability. Here, vividly, we see the intimate connection between emotional health and biological aging.

However, even amid these accumulating injuries, the body is far from helpless. Remarkably sophisticated defense systems work tirelessly behind the scenes, fighting biological decay. DNA repair enzymes mend damaged genetic material, robust antioxidant networks neutralize destructive ROS, and cellular recycling processes—like autophagy—diligently clear away harmful debris. Imagine these systems as tireless maintenance crews, continually repairing cellular damage and preserving our internal landscape. But even the most diligent workers eventually tire. With age, these protective mechanisms become less efficient, gradually overwhelmed by mounting damage. Eventually, the cumulative injuries surpass the body's ability to heal, culminating in the hallmark features of aging: weakened cellular function, compromised tissues, and diminished organ performance.

Understanding this interplay underscores a critical insight: aging is neither purely biological nor isolated in its causes. Rather, aging emerges from the dynamic interaction of genetic factors, metabolic processes, environmental exposures, and personal lifestyle decisions. Theories emphasizing oxidative damage, genetic instability, telomere shortening, and metabolic alterations do not stand apart; they form interconnected threads weaving a comprehensive, multidimensional picture of aging.

This interconnected understanding empowers us. By intentionally shaping our lifestyle choices—minimizing harmful environmental exposures, managing psychological stress, embracing nutritious diets, prioritizing regular physical activity, and ensuring restorative sleep—we gain substantial influence over our biological trajectory. Although we cannot pause time, we retain remarkable control over how time shapes our health.

Exploring these complex scientific narratives transforms our perception of aging. Viewing aging through the prism of cumulative damage and biological repair fosters a deeper respect for life's delicate balance, reminding us that while our choices shape our health profoundly, they unfold within nature's inescapable rhythms and boundaries.

The Cellular Senescence Theory: The Persistent Shadow of "Zombie" Cells

Every thriving city depends on careful upkeep—damaged buildings swiftly repaired, those beyond saving replaced. But when vigilance falters, decay quietly spreads, eroding the city's vitality piece by piece. Our bodies face a strikingly similar fate through cellular senescence: damaged cells cease dividing but refuse to leave, lingering silently in tissues. Early on, these so-called "zombie" cells act as protective guardians, diligently stopping the spread of potentially cancerous growths. Yet with age, their numbers multiply relentlessly, transforming from helpful sentinels into quiet saboteurs, steadily undermining the very tissues they once protected. Slowly, inconspicuously, these stubborn cells shift from guardians of health into quiet instigators of decline, casting a long shadow over our biological landscape.

The harmful impact of these tenacious cells emerges primarily from their secretion of a toxic brew known as the senescence-associated secretory phenotype (SASP). This inflammatory cocktail includes cytokines (molecules that ignite inflammation), chemokines (substances attracting inflammatory cells), and enzymes capable of degrading structural proteins. To visualize SASP's impact, consider your own skin. Over time, senescent fibroblasts significantly reduce their production of collagen—crucial for skin firmness and elasticity. Worse yet, they actively release enzymes that degrade existing collagen and elastin, accelerating the formation of wrinkles, sagging, and age spots. The mirror reflects these molecular realities: youthful elasticity gives way to deepening lines and lost firmness.

This destructive pattern repeats throughout the body. In arteries, the inflammatory effects of SASP contribute to vascular stiffening, compromised circulation, and elevated cardiovascular risk. Yet the disruption goes even deeper. Recent research uncovers a striking revelation: senescent cells don't merely remain passive nuisances; they actively eject fragments of damaged mitochondria—particularly mitochondrial DNA and double-stranded RNA—into surrounding tissues. Like tiny distress signals, these fragments trigger innate immune responses, fueling chronic, low-grade inflammation—a hallmark of aging that quietly undermines health from within.

Alarmingly, senescent cells can propagate their disruptive influence. Under certain conditions, their inflammatory signals induce neighboring healthy cells to enter senescence themselves, effectively recruiting new members into the ranks of cellular dysfunction. Although the speed and extent of this process vary across different tissues, its effect is undeniable—a self-sustaining cycle of inflammation, cellular decay, and cumulative harm.

Over time, this relentless accumulation of zombie cells significantly impairs immune function. The body's natural defenses weaken, diminishing its capacity to clear cellular debris, ward off infections, and respond robustly to stressors. Consider the brain, where senescent glial cells—accompanied by chronically activated microglia and astrocytes—fuel persistent neuroinflammation. Like static interfering with a clear radio signal, this inflammation disrupts neural communication, hastening cognitive decline and memory loss.

Cellular senescence thus embodies a striking biological paradox: beneficial during youth yet increasingly harmful with age. Recognizing this duality invites exciting possibilities. Could targeted removal or neutralization of these zombie cells help delay or even reverse aspects of age-related decline? If we envision these cells as the neglected buildings threatening our thriving biological city, the next step becomes clear: developing strategies to safely demolish or renovate them, restoring order, health, and vitality to our cellular neighborhoods.

The Cellular Impact of Glycation: Aging's Hidden Culprit

Think of a well-used kitchen sponge—initially flexible, absorbent, and resilient. Over time, however, repeated exposure to moisture, heat, and daily wear leaves it stiff, brittle, and less effective. Similarly, our bodies experience a quiet internal transformation through a process called glycation, slowly reshaping tissues from supple and flexible to stiffened and fragile. Glycation occurs when sugars chemically bind to proteins or fats, forming troublesome molecular complexes known as advanced glycation end-products (AGEs). These molecular "adhesives" quietly accumulate, steadily compromising cellular integrity, impairing tissue function, and fueling the persistent deterioration associated with aging.

The effects of glycation are both visibly apparent and internally disruptive. Externally, the skin provides a clear example. AGEs accumulate within the collagen fibers that grant youthful skin its supple elasticity, gradually stiffening these fibers until skin becomes less flexible and resilient. Picture someone noticing deepening wrinkles or sagging skin, not merely as superficial signs of age, but as outward signals of internal molecular stiffening. Beneath the surface, these once-flexible protein structures—collagen and elastin—lose their elasticity, manifesting externally as familiar signs of aging.

Internally, the impact extends deeper, quietly undermining cardiovascular health. Within arteries, glycation's molecular stickiness slowly but relentlessly diminishes the flexibility of vessel walls. Arteries stiffen, making it harder for blood to flow smoothly. Over the years, this slowly progressing rigidity increases blood pressure, places strain on the heart, and elevates the risk of cardiovascular disease. Much like pipes in an aging plumbing system becoming clogged and brittle, stiffened arteries compromise efficient blood flow and oxygen delivery, silently elevating disease risk.

In the brain, glycation operates like an unseen saboteur, contributing to neurodegenerative changes. AGEs facilitate the formation and stabilization of harmful protein clumps such as amyloid plaques and tau tangles—hallmarks of Alzheimer's disease. Think of these protein aggregates as tangled threads within a delicate tapestry, interrupting critical neural communication pathways and slowly dimming cognitive clarity. Over decades, the cumulative damage erodes memory, clarity, and cognitive agility, reflecting glycation's deeper, insidious influence.

Yet the rate and severity of glycation are highly responsive to our daily choices. Elevated blood sugar levels—often spurred by diets high in refined carbohydrates and sugars—dramatically accelerate AGE formation. Each sugary snack or highly processed meal potentially fuels microscopic processes that age the body faster. Fortunately, practical, intentional dietary adjustments offer significant protective potential. Reducing refined sugars, choosing balanced nutrition rich in antioxidants, and maintaining stable blood glucose levels can substantially limit AGE formation and slow structural and functional damage. These choices, made consistently over time, offer real pathways toward healthier aging.

Scientists, equipped with deeper insights into glycation's intricate molecular mechanisms, now actively pursue strategies to mitigate its harmful effects. Current research explores promising interventions, from pharmaceutical approaches designed to prevent AGE formation, to lifestyle-based strategies that enhance the body's natural AGE-clearance abilities. Could controlling glycation represent a pivotal step toward influencing how we age—shifting aging from a passive inevitability to an active, manageable process? An intriguing question.

Understanding glycation empowers us, transforming aging from a passive experience of decline into an active, intentional narrative. With this deeper knowledge, aging no longer signifies the ticking clock of biological fate; rather, it becomes a story we can shape—a process enriched by deliberate, informed decisions. Recognizing glycation's inconspicuous yet widespread effects underscores the importance of continued scientific research—not solely for groundbreaking discoveries, but because even incremental advances can lead to practical improvements in health and quality of life as we age.

The Genetic and Epigenetic Theories of Aging: Decoding Longevity's Blueprint and Dynamic Expression

Within every living cell lies DNA, an elegant molecular blueprint that orchestrates life's most fundamental processes—growth and healing, adaptation and resilience. According to the Genetic Theory of Aging, certain genes associated with longevity serve as biological caretakers, diligently maintaining cellular integrity, optimizing metabolism, and fortifying the body against stress. Yet genes never operate in isolation; instead, they participate in intricate networks, collectively influencing our body's remarkable capacity to repair itself, sustain equilibrium, and navigate the accumulating wear of time.

THE ART, SCIENCE, AND STRATEGY OF LONGEVITY

Genetic inheritance varies considerably from one person to another, deeply influencing each person's unique path of aging. Some people inherit beneficial genetic variants—quiet biological blessings that bolster DNA repair, fine-tune metabolism, and enhance resistance to chronic diseases. Others carry genetic vulnerabilities: mutations or less favorable gene variants that compromise cellular repair, disrupt stress-response pathways, and accelerate age-related decline. But genes alone never write our aging story in isolation. Instead, aging emerges through a dynamic dialogue between inherited genetic potential and the external influences of environment and lifestyle. Choices involving nutrition, physical activity, stress management, and environmental exposures continuously shape how our genetic potential unfolds, guiding whether we fully realize the longevity encoded in our genes.

Building upon this genetic foundation, the Epigenetic Theory of Aging offers a more nuanced perspective on how gene expression dynamically evolves throughout a lifetime. If DNA serves as life's foundational script, then epigenetics acts as an interpreter—carefully deciding precisely when genes awaken or fall silent. Epigenetic regulation occurs through chemical modifications, primarily DNA methylation (chemical tags that attach directly to DNA and guide gene activity) and histone acetylation (which influences how tightly DNA is wrapped and thus how readily genes can be accessed). These chemical adjustments don't alter the genetic code itself; instead, they finely tune gene expression in response to our internal physiological state, daily behaviors, and environmental exposures.

Over decades, however, this precise epigenetic choreography begins to falter, leading to what scientists aptly call "epigenetic drift." Beneficial genes essential for repairing cells, regulating inflammation, and maintaining metabolic efficiency may become mistakenly silenced, while harmful genes associated with chronic inflammation or tissue deterioration awaken and intensify. Gradually, this loss of epigenetic precision erodes cellular function, weakens immune defenses, and reduces regenerative capacity—hallmarks of biological aging silently unfolding beneath the surface.

Importantly, epigenetic drift is neither inevitable nor fixed. Because epigenetic patterns remain inherently responsive, they offer exciting therapeutic opportunities for influencing aging directly. Current research actively explores ways to reset these molecular markers, potentially reversing aspects of age-related decline. Could future interventions restore our cells' youthful precision, reshaping the trajectory of aging? A question that needs to be answered.

At the forefront of these developments stand epigenetic clocks—innovative tools that measure biological age by analyzing patterns of DNA methylation. Unlike chronological age, which simply counts birthdays, biological age reflects our actual physiological health at the cellular level. Two people with identical chronological ages can display strikingly different biological profiles, influenced significantly by genetics, diet quality, physical activity, stress levels, and exposure to environmental toxins. Epigenetic clocks interpret these molecular fingerprints, offering a personalized snapshot of biological aging.

The practical implications of epigenetic clocks are profound. By revealing molecular indicators of accelerated or slowed aging, scientists can precisely determine which lifestyle choices or therapeutic interventions effectively extend healthspan. Epigenetic clocks thus become active tools—not merely passive measurements—guiding personalized interventions designed to reshape aging.

Recent breakthroughs in non-invasive epigenetic testing have greatly increased the accessibility of biological age assessments. Simple techniques, like cheek swabs or saliva samples, now enable regular tracking of epigenetic markers without invasive blood draws or complicated procedures. This convenience greatly enhances longitudinal research, allowing frequent, real-world monitoring of molecular aging markers over extended periods.

Moreover, innovative tissue-specific epigenetic clocks offer even greater precision, unveiling unique aging patterns across distinct tissues and organs. Cells in the liver, brain neurons, heart tissue, and immune system age at differing rates, highlighting the complexity and variability of aging's progression. Understanding these delicate variations allows researchers to craft interventions carefully tailored to the most vulnerable tissues—whether protecting cognitive clarity, strengthening cardiovascular health, or enhancing immune function.

Uncovering the intricate dance between genetics and epigenetics transforms our fundamental understanding of aging. No longer viewed as predetermined genetic fate nor only environmental consequence, aging emerges as a vibrant, ongoing dialogue between inherited potential and daily experience. This rich interplay explains how two people with similar genetic backgrounds can follow dramatically different aging journeys. Every choice—dietary habits, physical activity, stress management, sleep quality, and social connection—sends epigenetic signals, shaping gene expression powerfully and persistently.

Integrating these insights fundamentally alters how we approach aging. Longevity becomes not just inherited potential but an empowering opportunity, a deeply personal narrative shaped by informed decisions, purposeful actions, and the emerging science of epigenetics. Aging thus ceases to represent inevitable decline and instead unfolds as a story we consciously influence—a story filled with resilience, intentionality, and genuine human flourishing.

Aging, in short, is not destiny. It is dialogue.

The Mitochondrial Theory: Aging's Energy Crisis

At the heart of every living cell are mitochondria—tiny, tireless structures often described as cellular powerhouses. Like miniature factories humming constantly, they produce adenosine triphosphate (ATP), the indispensable energy currency that fuels virtually all biological activities. Yet this continuous energy production comes at an inevitable price. While generating ATP, mitochondria simultaneously produce reactive oxygen species (ROS)—highly unstable molecules that behave like microscopic sparks, capable of igniting damage within critical cellular components such as proteins, lipid membranes, and mitochondrial DNA (mtDNA).

Early in life, robust antioxidant defenses swiftly extinguish these ROS "sparks," protecting cells from oxidative harm and maintaining their internal harmony. As decades pass, however, these antioxidant mechanisms gradually diminish, allowing oxidative damage to relentlessly build. Mitochondrial DNA is especially vulnerable; situated close to the ROS-generating sites and equipped with limited repair capabilities, it slowly collects irreversible injuries. This gradual accumulation triggers a damaging cycle: injured mitochondria produce less ATP while paradoxically increasing their output of ROS, fueling a downward spiral of cellular dysfunction.

Nowhere is mitochondrial impairment more vividly felt than in energy-demanding tissues. Consider the brain, a dynamic organ constantly craving fuel. Here, mitochondrial dysfunction undermines neural health, accelerating cognitive decline and leaving the brain increasingly vulnerable to diseases like Alzheimer's and Parkinson's. Similarly, within the heart—a muscle tirelessly contracting billions of times throughout a lifetime—reduced mitochondrial efficiency gradually weakens cardiac strength and increases susceptibility to heart disease. Skeletal muscles, too, experience mitochondrial decline, manifesting as sarcopenia: the slow, insidious loss of muscle mass and strength. Over time, this reduces mobility, independence, and overall quality of life.

Mitochondria do far more than produce energy. They also participate actively in cell signaling, regulating cell death (apoptosis), and managing oxidative stress. As mitochondrial function falters, these essential regulatory roles suffer, disrupting cellular balance and amplifying aging's impact across the body's interconnected systems.

Given their critical role in aging, mitochondria have become a major focus of longevity research. Scientists are actively exploring targeted strategies—from caloric restriction, fasting, and mitochondrial-specific antioxidants to innovative pharmacological and biotechnological interventions—to protect and rejuvenate mitochondrial health. By combining lifestyle adjustments with targeted therapies, longevity science aims not only to extend lifespan but to sustain vitality, resilience, and meaningful independence across our additional years. Aging thus becomes less an inevitable decline, and more an engaging quest—one that empowers us to protect, nurture, and restore the cellular foundations of life.

The Inflammation Theory: Aging's Quiet Fire

Beneath the calm surface of the body simmers a silent yet persistent fire—one faint enough to remain unnoticed, yet fierce enough to gradually erode health over decades. Scientists have termed this chronic internal smoldering "inflammaging," a condition characterized by steady, low-level inflammation deeply embedded in the aging process. Unlike acute inflammation—the body's rapid, protective response to injury or infection—inflammaging insidiously endures, continuously taxing cells and tissues, slowly unraveling biological resilience.

Multiple forces feed this chronic fire. Central among them are senescent cells, those biological "zombies" that no longer divide but stubbornly persist. Though dormant, these cells are hardly silent. As previously discussed, they secrete an inflammatory mix known as the senescence-associated secretory phenotype (SASP)—a biochemical brew of molecules that acts like signals leaping to surrounding healthy cells, triggering inflammatory responses. Through these signaling molecules, senescent cells recruit healthy neighbors into their dysfunctional state, perpetuating a self-sustaining cycle of cellular distress.

Oxidative stress further fuels the flames. Reactive oxygen species (ROS), described earlier in mitochondrial function, contribute significantly to chronic inflammation. This oxidative damage accumulates steadily, provoking immune cells into action and intensifying the inflammatory cycle. The body finds itself locked in a constant internal struggle, caught in an exhausting loop: damage fuels inflammation, inflammation generates more damage, and the cycle continues relentlessly.

Even our gut microbiome—the vibrant community of microorganisms residing within our digestive tract—plays a crucial role. With age, the once-diverse microbiome tends toward imbalance, shifting away from beneficial microbes and toward harmful bacterial species. Concurrently, the intestinal barrier weakens, a condition popularly known as "leaky gut syndrome." This porous lining allows microbial toxins to leak into the bloodstream, prompting an ongoing, low-grade immune reaction that continuously stokes systemic inflammation.

The consequences ripple widely, affecting organs from skin to brain. Within arteries, persistent inflammation, while imperceptible, hardens vessel walls, raising blood pressure and increasing heart disease risk. In the brain, chronic inflammation gradually impairs neural function, heightening susceptibility to cognitive impairment and neurodegenerative conditions. Even the immune system itself gradually weakens, worn down by decades of persistent, low-level activation—its protective vigilance slowly replaced by vulnerability.

With greater understanding comes the power of proactive intervention. Researchers now explore targeted ways to douse the flames of inflammaging, from anti-inflammatory dietary patterns rich in antioxidants and omega-3 fatty acids to lifestyle strategies like regular exercise, meditation, and quality sleep. Pharmacological interventions targeting inflammatory pathways hold promising potential, alongside exciting new therapies designed to rebalance the microbiome and restore intestinal integrity. Emerging microbiome modulation techniques and innovative senolytic treatments offer tantalizing opportunities to neutralize inflammaging at its source.

In embracing these scientific insights, aging transforms from passive inevitability into an active and empowering narrative. Rather than passively accepting the quiet inflammation smoldering within, people can actively influence their biological trajectory. Understanding the underlying mechanisms of inflammaging reveals aging as a biologically modifiable process, highlighting valuable opportunities for early intervention to slow the progression of age-related decline.

The Telomere Shortening Theory: Aging's Cellular Countdown

Within each cell resides DNA—life's precious instruction manual—protected at its ends by specialized molecular "caps" known as telomeres. Often likened to the plastic tips on shoelaces that prevent fraying, telomeres steadily shorten each time a cell divides, gradually losing their protective ability. Eventually, telomeres reach a critical length, signaling cells that their healthy lifespan is near an end. At this crossroads, cells either enter senescence—a dormant, dysfunctional state reminiscent of cellular zombies—or undergo apoptosis, a precisely choreographed cellular self-destruction.

Telomere attrition reveals itself vividly in tissues characterized by rapid and continual regeneration, such as our immune system and digestive tract. Consider immune cells, essential defenders against infections and illness. Early in life, ample telomere length supports robust immune responses, enabling rapid cell proliferation and effective defense. Yet as years accumulate and telomeres shorten, immune cell regeneration falters, quietly weakening our defenses and heightening susceptibility to infections and chronic conditions. Similarly, the lining of our gut—dependent on constant renewal to ensure efficient digestion and nutrient absorption—gradually deteriorates, diminishing digestive function and overall nutritional health. In both cases, internal cellular aging insidiously undermines critical functions, progressively eroding vitality and health from within.

Still, telomeres do more than track time's passage—they actively and directly shape the pace of aging. Intriguingly, our daily choices materially influence telomere length. Chronic stress, diets rich in refined sugars, and sedentary lifestyles accelerate telomere erosion, hastening biological aging at the cellular level. By contrast, balanced nutrition, regular physical activity, intentional stress management, and meaningful social connections slow telomere loss, effectively preserving cellular resilience. The power to influence our telomere length—and thus our healthspan—is literally within our grasp.

Remarkably, researchers have begun harnessing this biological insight, exploring interventions designed to protect or even lengthen telomeres. Emerging therapeutic strategies—such as pharmacological compounds, lifestyle interventions, or innovative treatments stimulating telomerase (the enzyme that rebuilds telomeres)—promise to extend not just lifespan but the vitality and quality of life. Recent studies reveal encouraging possibilities, prompting the question: Could therapies targeting telomere preservation hold the key to delaying age-related diseases and restoring tissue function in later years?

Understanding telomere biology transforms aging from a passive acceptance of fate into an empowering narrative of choice. Rather than simply marking the passage of biological time, telomeres serve as dynamic indicators—reflecting the intricate balance among genetics, environmental influences, and intentional actions. Studying these molecular structures reveals the interplay between inherent biological limits and scientific advances capable of reshaping or even extending cellular boundaries.

The Neuroendocrine Theory: Aging's Hormonal Symphony

At the core of aging lies a delicate biological symphony—a harmonious interplay of hormones masterfully conducted by the brain's hypothalamus. In youth, this intricate hormonal orchestra performs flawlessly, synchronizing metabolism, growth, stress responses, reproduction, and tissue repair into a unified, resilient whole. Yet, over decades, the precision of this hormonal symphony gently fades, gradually slipping into imbalance. Melodies that once flowed effortlessly become discordant, contributing significantly to the body's progressive decline.

Consider growth hormone, a key player in tissue regeneration, muscle vitality, and skin elasticity. In our younger years, abundant growth hormone maintains robust tissues—muscles repair swiftly, skin stays firm, and bones remain strong. But with aging, its production diminishes like a slowly fading musical note, and the body's regenerative vigor wanes. Muscles weaken, wounds heal more slowly, skin becomes thinner and fragile, and bones grow porous and brittle.

Similarly, estrogen and testosterone—vital reproductive hormones—decline over time, casting their own shadows over our health. As these hormones ebb, cognitive clarity dims, bones lose density, and cardiovascular strength falters. The steady hormonal harmony of youth gradually gives way to imbalance, slowly eroding our resilience from within.

Adding complexity to this hormonal symphony is cortisol, the body's primary stress hormone. Normally, cortisol serves as a powerful protector in short bursts, preparing us for action or alertness. But as we age, cortisol levels often linger chronically elevated, a once-helpful melody now echoing continuously, overwhelming the biological orchestra. This persistent high cortisol triggers ongoing inflammation, weakens immune defenses, clouds cognitive sharpness, and accelerates cellular aging—transforming a beneficial short-term response into a chronic detriment.

This unraveling of hormonal harmony need not be inevitable. Tailored hormone replacement therapies, carefully combined with lifestyle practices such as balanced nutrition, regular exercise, mindful stress management, and quality sleep, can significantly delay or even reverse hormonal imbalances. Through intentional, informed actions, we become active participants—conductors ourselves—in our body's hormonal performance. This proactive approach helps sustain physical strength, cognitive clarity, emotional balance, and lasting vitality, transforming biological decline into a dynamic, manageable journey. It invites us to recognize our power to influence the body's intricate hormonal melodies, actively shaping the quality and vibrancy of our extended years. This perspective emphasizes that aging involves complex hormonal interactions, reminding us that preserving health with age relies not on chasing eternal youth, but on carefully sustaining balance within our body's intricate biological networks.

IOULIA HOWARD AND DON HOWARD

The Disposable Soma Theory: Evolution's Delicate Balancing Act

Why would evolution, so tirelessly focused on refining life for survival, allow organisms to age? The Disposable Soma Theory provides an insightful answer: aging isn't a biological oversight but a carefully calibrated compromise shaped by resource constraints. Life faces a perpetual balancing act between allocating limited energy resources toward reproduction—the essential task of passing genes to future generations—and preserving bodily integrity (the soma) through continuous maintenance and repair.

This evolutionary bargain plays out vividly across the natural world. Take mice, for instance—tiny creatures racing against time, investing furiously in rapid reproduction. They produce multiple litters in quick succession, channeling their energy into offspring rather than long-term self-preservation. The consequence? Their lifespan is fleeting, a brief spark quickly extinguished once reproductive tasks are complete. Humans, whales, and other long-lived species, by contrast, initially dedicate substantial energy toward meticulous bodily upkeep, allowing extended reproductive opportunities and better odds of survival. Yet even among these species, this commitment to cellular maintenance inevitably fades. As reproductive potential wanes, evolution quietly withdraws its investment in bodily repair, accelerating the aging process.

Viewing aging as this evolutionary negotiation transforms how we understand our biological journey. Aging isn't nature's flaw—it's a logical consequence of life's pragmatic strategy to favor reproduction and genetic legacy over endless physical upkeep. Yet recognizing the rules of this ancient compromise grants us a measure of agency: if resource allocation shapes aging, perhaps we can strategically intervene.

Practical actions—including intentional dietary choices, regular physical activity, deliberate stress reduction, and innovative scientific therapies—can positively influence this delicate evolutionary balance. By consciously directing resources toward bodily maintenance and repair, we shift from passive observers to active contributors in shaping our aging experience.

Yet even as we adopt these strategies, aging remains inherently complex, influenced not only by our individual decisions but also by genetics, environmental factors, and the uncertainties embedded within life.

Mosaic of Time: Weaving Biology, Complexity, and Purpose

Aging is not just a biological progression or a passive drift toward inevitable frailty; it is a complex narrative artfully pieced into the mosaic of human existence—a meaningful and multidimensional journey. During youth, sophisticated biological mechanisms sustain vitality, ensuring cellular integrity and robust health. Over time, however, imperceptible shifts occur; protective processes gradually diminish, tipping the body's balance toward vulnerability and dysfunction.

Genetic blueprints, epigenetic modifications, metabolic rhythms, and cellular defenses do not operate in isolation; instead, they continually interact, dynamically sculpting one another. Aging can be envisioned as an intricate ecosystem, composed of diverse biological elements—each playing an essential role yet progressively shifting or declining over time. Individually, these elements hold significance; collectively, however, their interactions reveal the complexity of aging and the gradual transformations unfolding within us as the years advance.

This biological dynamic remains highly responsive to intervention. Aging is not a fixed destiny dictated solely by genetics—it is an evolving narrative guided by deliberate choices. How we age is remarkably pliable—influenced by what we eat, how we move, the calm we cultivate, the depth of our sleep, and the medical insights we choose to embrace.

With this understanding, aging shifts from passive acceptance to an active pursuit. It invites resilience, meaningful connections, and deeper engagement with life's broader purpose. Aging becomes a dialogue between biology and intention, where conscious choices continually shape and enrich our experience.

Part II

The Foundations of Longevity—Proven Strategies for a Healthier, Longer Life

Aging represents more than the accumulation of years; it is the ongoing refinement of life—a dynamic journey continually altered by our daily choices and actions. Modern science reveals aging as an adaptable and responsive process, influenced by our decisions regarding movement, nutrition, rest, stress management, and social connections. Each choice affects whether we progress toward sustained health or gradual deterioration.

Movement, for instance, serves as a daily affirmation of autonomy and vigor. Beyond simple exercise, regular physical engagement sustains muscle integrity, bone density, and cognitive sharpness, safeguarding our independence. Similarly, nutrition transcends basic sustenance, promoting cellular repair, reducing inflammation, and enhancing overall energy. Sleep—often undervalued—replenishes the body and mind incrementally, enhancing cognitive clarity, immune robustness, and emotional balance. Stress management complements these pillars by anchoring us amid life's inevitable uncertainties, cultivating psychological composure and physiological stability.

Genuine longevity depends on foundations deeper than physical well-being alone. Comprehensive wellness integrates emotional adaptability, spiritual enrichment, and meaningful social bonds. Relationships characterized by intimacy, friendship, and companionship infuse life with purpose and depth, ensuring that advancing years are measured not by duration but by authentic shared experiences. Intentional connections thus elevate growing older from survival into enrichment.

In the chapters ahead, we will move beyond theoretical understanding to explore practical pathways—revealing how movement restores robustness, nutrition sustains vitality, and mindful decisions coupled with emotional wellness enhance the quality of life. Aging, in this light, is no longer a predetermined decline but an evolving narrative, consciously shaped through insight and intention.

By embracing this empowering perspective, we reclaim agency over our experience of aging. Life deepens, and each year becomes not something to endure, but an opportunity—an invitation to cultivate strength, nurture emotional resilience, and engage with ourselves and others. Perhaps the greatest reward of aging lies not in meticulously orchestrating every moment but in appreciating life's quieter rhythms—the subtle, unspoken moments that unite us in our shared humanity.

CHAPTER 4

Movement is Medicine—The Power of Physical Activity

"The journey of a thousand miles begins with a single step."
—Lao Tzu

One practice holds extraordinary power to strengthen the heart, sharpen the mind, and extend both healthspan and lifespan—movement. Far more fundamental than a fitness tool or transient health trend, regular physical activity is a biological imperative embedded within our physiology. At the cellular level, movement triggers transformative processes, sustaining vitality and preserving functional independence across decades.

Exercise goes well beyond calorie burning and muscle building; it activates potent cellular repair mechanisms, regulates inflammation, and fortifies critical systems against the ravages of aging. Maintaining mobility, flexibility, and strength ensures that aging need not equate to weakness. Instead, it can mean preserving autonomy, safeguarding physical capability, and fully participating in everyday life. Each walk, stretch, or resistance-training session reinforces resilience, delays frailty, and enriches quality of life.

Movement's influence surpasses the physical, benefiting mental and emotional well-being. Physical activity enhances cognitive function, promotes neuroplasticity—the brain's remarkable ability to adapt and reorganize—and reduces the risk of neurodegenerative conditions such as Alzheimer's disease. An active body supports an active mind. Those who move regularly tend to experience greater clarity, creativity, and emotional stability throughout their lives.

Scientific evidence confirms unequivocally: consistent movement optimizes cardiovascular health, strengthens bones and joints, enhances metabolic function, and reduces the risk of heart disease, diabetes, and certain cancers. Movement is not only preventive—it actively renews and revitalizes nearly every dimension of human health.

The first step is simple: choose to move. Whether taking stairs instead of elevators, walking in nature, gardening, or engaging in basic strength-building exercises, every motion counts. Movement is more than medicine—it fosters freedom, builds resilience, and provides the foundation for maintaining an active, independent life.

The Evolutionary Perspective—Why Humans Are Designed for Movement

Human beings are not only capable of movement; we are biologically designed for it. Unlike species whose survival relies on brief bursts of speed or raw power, humans evolved predominantly for endurance. Our ancestors did not chase prey with rapid sprints; instead, they utilized "persistence hunting," patiently tracking animals over vast distances until exhaustion left prey unable to escape. This sustained physical effort shaped our physiology profoundly—from cardiovascular efficiency and muscular structure to metabolic flexibility.

Human anatomy reflects these adaptations explicitly. Long limbs, upright posture, and efficient sweat glands for cooling enable us to sustain physical exertion without overheating. Predominantly slow-twitch muscle fibers conserve energy, supporting stamina over extended periods. Collectively, these evolutionary traits underscore a fundamental truth: consistent movement is essential to human health.

This critical relationship between habitual movement and longevity is evident in contemporary examples of exceptional aging. "Blue Zones"—regions with notably high concentrations of centenarians—demonstrate how routine, integrated physical activity contributes significantly to sustained vitality. Populations in places like Okinawa, Japan, and Sardinia, Italy, naturally embed movement into their everyday lives through long walks, gardening, and manual labor. This continuous physical activity safeguards musculoskeletal and cardiovascular health while dramatically reducing chronic disease risk.

Modern lifestyles, however, often distance us from our evolutionary blueprint. Prolonged sitting, reliance on motorized transportation, and reduced physical labor have disrupted our natural connection to movement, fueling metabolic disorders, cardiovascular diseases, and frailty. Yet research consistently affirms that incorporating regular, moderate physical activities—ranging from leisure pursuits to structured fitness routines—can effectively restore physiological balance and support healthy aging.

Movement, therefore, is not simply a lifestyle choice; it is a biological necessity for preserving health and longevity.

The Science of Movement: How Exercise Fuels Longevity

Exercise extends beyond physical fitness; it acts as a powerful biological catalyst, initiating cellular adaptations that significantly influence longevity. By enhancing energy production, genetic regulation, and cellular resilience, movement directly impacts core elements of the aging process, substantially extending healthspan.

One primary way exercise supports longevity is through mitochondrial biogenesis—the creation of new mitochondria, cellular "powerhouses" that produce energy (ATP). Central to this process is AMPK (adenosine monophosphate-activated protein kinase), an enzyme that senses cellular energy availability. During exercise, temporary energy depletion activates AMPK, prompting mitochondria production to restore energy equilibrium. Over time, mitochondria naturally lose effectiveness, contributing to fatigue and increasing susceptibility to age-related diseases. Regular physical activity counters this decline, bolstering mitochondrial efficiency, improving glucose metabolism, enhancing insulin sensitivity, and reducing the risk of diabetes, cardiovascular disease, and neurodegenerative disorders.

Aging also involves balancing tissue growth and repair—a delicate equilibrium influenced significantly by exercise. Physical activity modulates two critical yet opposing biological pathways: mTOR (mechanistic target of rapamycin), a central cellular pathway that regulates growth, repair, and protein synthesis, and autophagy, the body's internal recycling system that degrades and removes damaged proteins, organelles, and other cellular components—supporting cellular renewal and metabolic homeostasis. Resistance training activates mTOR, stimulating muscle growth, tissue repair, and protein synthesis—processes vital for preserving muscle mass and strength, both of which decline with age. However, excessive nutrient availability and inactivity can cause mTOR to remain persistently active, suppressing autophagy. Aerobic exercise and intermittent fasting stimulate autophagy, supporting cellular renewal and reducing toxic protein buildup associated with conditions such as Alzheimer's and Parkinson's diseases. Thus, regular movement maintains the body's flexibility, resilience, and regenerative capacity.

Additionally, exercise preserves cellular integrity through enhanced proteostasis—the maintenance of healthy protein functions within cells. Misfolded or damaged proteins can accumulate, disrupting cellular health and accelerating aging. Exercise activates heat shock proteins, molecular "chaperones" that repair or clear misfolded proteins before harmful aggregations form. This mechanism is particularly crucial for preventing neurodegenerative diseases, which are characterized by harmful protein clusters.

Physical activity further influences gene expression through epigenetic mechanisms. Though the genetic code remains stable, exercise fine-tunes gene activity via DNA methylation and histone modification. These alterations activate protective genes and silence harmful ones, reducing inflammation, oxidative stress, and metabolic dysfunction—all significant drivers of aging.

At its core, movement is more than exercise—it is a biological inheritance, encoded through millennia of adaptation. When we engage this primal rhythm, we go beyond preserving function; we recalibrate aging itself, exchanging drift for direction and passivity for purposeful motion.

Inflammation and Oxidative Stress: Exercise as a Natural Regulator

As explored in depth in a previous chapter, chronic low-grade inflammation accelerates aging, fueling a cascade of conditions ranging from cardiovascular disease and arthritis to neurodegeneration and metabolic dysfunction. Although acute inflammation is beneficial and necessary—swiftly healing wounds such as a scraped knee through precise immune responses—persistent inflammation acts more like a smoldering fire, steadily eroding cellular health and leaving tissues increasingly vulnerable to disease.

Fortunately, regular physical activity serves as a powerful natural countermeasure by naturally recalibrating the body's inflammatory signaling pathways. Exercise significantly reduces harmful pro-inflammatory cytokines, such as tumor necrosis factor-alpha (TNF-α) and interleukin-6 (IL-6), while simultaneously enhancing beneficial anti-inflammatory mediators, notably interleukin-10 (IL-10). This elegant balance curtails chronic tissue damage, boosts immune efficiency, and fortifies systemic resilience, helping protect the body against the gradual toll of age-related disease.

In addition to its anti-inflammatory effects, exercise remarkably refines our body's defenses against oxidative stress—a creeping but persistent biochemical phenomenon analogous to rust accumulating within our cells. Initially, physical activity briefly elevates reactive oxygen species (ROS), highly reactive molecules capable of damaging cellular structures. Yet this seemingly paradoxical increase triggers hormesis—a beneficial adaptive response that strengthens intrinsic antioxidant defenses. With consistent exercise, our bodies produce more powerful antioxidants like superoxide dismutase (SOD) and glutathione, which diligently neutralize free radicals and minimize oxidative harm. Thus, periodic, moderate exercise-induced stress cultivates enduring cellular resilience, positioning physical activity as a natural guardian against aging, oxidative damage, and chronic illness.

This interplay between inflammation and oxidative stress directly contributes to cellular aging by promoting the shortening of telomeres, which protect chromosome ends from damage. With each cell division, telomeres erode, eventually driving cells into senescence. Regular exercise slows this attrition by reducing inflammation and oxidative stress, preserving cellular integrity and sustaining the body's regenerative capacity.

Moreover, exercise proactively engages the body's regenerative mechanisms by activating tissue-specific stem cells. Satellite cells nestled within muscles promptly mobilize with physical exertion, facilitating muscle repair and regeneration. Similarly, neural progenitor cells within the brain respond to regular movement, promoting neuroplasticity and enhancing tissue renewal. By nurturing these vital stem cell populations, consistent physical activity counters age-related tissue deterioration—preserving strength, adaptability, and the body's capacity to recover throughout the shifting seasons of life.

In essence, exercise surpasses isolated effects—it masterfully coordinates an expansive network of biological processes to slow aging, reinforce resilience, and extend our healthspan. By optimizing mitochondrial efficiency, harmonizing cellular growth and repair, protecting telomere integrity, managing inflammation, and encouraging robust cellular renewal, physical activity emerges as a holistic strategy against aging. Its integrated benefits reinforce the body's structural harmony, softening time's impact and preserving the intricate elegance of human health.

Exercise and Whole-Body Health: Strengthening Every System

Exercise is one of the most potent and versatile interventions available for preventing disease, benefiting nearly every physiological system in the body. By enhancing resilience, restoring internal balance, and diminishing the risks of chronic conditions, regular physical activity serves as a foundational catalyst for long-term health.

Unlike pharmaceutical approaches, which often isolate single diseases or symptoms, exercise awakens a vast, interconnected network of biological mechanisms. Movement fortifies the heart, optimizes metabolic function, reinforces immune defenses, and safeguards cognitive abilities, making it a universally accessible, life-affirming strategy against aging-related diseases. Consistent physical activity creates a biological environment in which each system of the body can perform optimally—allowing movement to become our strongest protection against physical decline and disease.

Strengthening the Heart and Circulatory System

A robust cardiovascular system stands as the cornerstone of longevity, and exercise plays a foundational role in its maintenance. Each time the heart contracts during physical exertion, the cardiac muscle strengthens incrementally, enhancing its capacity to pump blood efficiently throughout the body. This repeated stimulation lowers blood pressure, improves arterial elasticity, and dramatically reduces the risk of hypertension, stroke, and heart disease—the leading cause of death worldwide. Imagine arteries as flexible garden hoses, effortlessly transporting nutrients and oxygen; exercise helps keep these blood vessels supple, responsive, and free from plaque accumulation.

Even modest amounts of physical activity yield profound, life-extending benefits. Studies consistently demonstrate that short bouts of vigorous movement—such as brisk walking, energetic cycling, or focused resistance training—can reduce cardiovascular mortality by up to 50%. By optimizing cardiovascular efficiency, regular movement ensures that tissues receive essential nutrients and oxygen more effectively, supporting cellular vitality, sustaining energy levels, and significantly lowering the risk of life-threatening cardiac events. With each heartbeat enhanced through regular physical activity, the body becomes increasingly resilient, adaptable, and prepared for the ongoing demands of aging.

Regulating Metabolism and Preventing Diabetes

Beyond its cardiovascular benefits, exercise serves as an essential pillar of metabolic health, offering robust protection against diabetes, obesity, and insulin resistance. In sedentary individuals, insulin—the hormone that regulates blood sugar—becomes less effective, increasing the risk of type 2 diabetes and broader metabolic dysfunction. Regular physical movement sensitizes muscle cells to insulin, improving glucose uptake, reducing excessive insulin demand, and helping maintain stable blood sugar levels—like fine-tuning an intricate biological thermostat.

Aerobic exercises, such as jogging or swimming, and resistance training, like weightlifting, provide distinct yet synergistic metabolic benefits. Extensive research shows that consistent physical activity significantly lowers fasting glucose levels and reduces hemoglobin A1c—a key long-term marker for diabetes risk. Moreover, exercise prevents the dangerous accumulation of excess fat, especially visceral fat around vital organs, which is closely linked to chronic systemic inflammation, cardiovascular disease, and metabolic syndrome.

Maintaining energy balance, optimizing glucose metabolism, and lowering inflammatory markers, regular movement serves as a frontline defense against metabolic diseases, reinforcing lasting health and resilience. Aging need not signify inevitable metabolic decline. With every step walked, weight lifted, and gentle stretch performed, the body continuously renews its extraordinary capacity to regulate energy, ward off disease, and maintain durable physical resilience across a lifetime.

Defending Against Cancer and Strengthening Immunity

Exercise also emerges as a formidable ally in cancer prevention, fortifying immune function and regulating complex biological pathways involved in tumor development. Each session of physical activity mobilizes immune sentinels—natural killer (NK) cells, macrophages, and T cells—that diligently patrol the body, identifying and neutralizing abnormal cells before they transform into malignant tumors. It is as if exercise trains a vigilant army within, primed to detect and eliminate threats swiftly and efficiently.

Research repeatedly links regular physical activity to significantly reduced incidences of breast, colon, and prostate cancers. Movement helps modulate hormone levels, diminish systemic inflammation, and enhance DNA repair mechanisms, safeguarding genetic integrity. Moreover, exercise positively influences tumor-suppressing genes, strengthening the body's innate defenses against potential cancerous growths. By boosting immune efficiency and simultaneously counteracting chronic inflammation—two major contributors to cancer progression—exercise stands as an exceptional, non-pharmacological strategy for cancer prevention.

Preserving Musculoskeletal Health and Preventing Frailty

Strong muscles and healthy bones form the foundation for long-term mobility, independence, and overall well-being, and exercise offers an essential means of maintaining both. As the years pass, sarcopenia—the gradual, age-related loss of muscle mass and strength—becomes increasingly common, heightening risks for frailty, falls, and metabolic dysfunction. Picture an older adult confidently climbing stairs or gracefully carrying groceries, contrasted with someone weakened by unchecked muscle loss; the difference often lies in regular strength training. By stimulating muscle protein synthesis, preserving fast-twitch (type II) muscle fibers crucial for quick reactions, and enhancing neuromuscular coordination, strength exercises promote balance, mobility, and responsive movement throughout life.

The benefits extend beyond muscles alone, as bones also thrive with regular physical activity. Resistance training and weight-bearing activities—such as lifting weights or brisk walking—actively stimulate osteoblasts, the specialized cells responsible for building and maintaining bone density. These exercises fortify bones against osteoporosis and significantly reduce the likelihood of fractures. Everyday movements, including walking, running, or resistance exercises, not only sustain skeletal strength but also stabilize joints, enhance posture, and preserve functional movement. Collectively, these activities safeguard against falls and nurture independence, helping us remain active, physically confident, and self-reliant even into advanced age.

Enhancing Gut Health and the Microbiome

Emerging research continues to illuminate the fascinating connection between regular exercise and gut health, underscoring how physical movement enriches microbial diversity, strengthens digestion, and moderates inflammation. The gut microbiome—an intricate community of trillions of microorganisms—plays a central role in immune function, nutrient absorption, and overall metabolic health. Studies consistently demonstrate that physical activity increases populations of beneficial bacteria, particularly those producing short-chain fatty acids (SCFAs). Like nurturing a lush, vibrant garden within, these beneficial microbes reinforce gut-barrier integrity, regulate immune responses, and dampen systemic inflammation, positioning exercise as a comprehensive intervention that extends well beyond traditional metabolic benefits.

Remarkably, the beneficial relationship between the gut and exercise reaches even further, influencing the brain through the gut-brain axis—a dynamic communication channel linking digestive health with emotional well-being, cognitive function, and stress resilience. Physical activity positively modulates this complex interplay, fostering a more diverse and balanced microbiome that, in turn, contributes to neurological function and mental well-being. Thus, regular movement not only improves digestion and immunity but also enhances mood stability and cognitive performance. This rich triad of exercise, gut health, and brain function underscores the deep interconnection between movement, mental vitality, and long-term health.

Exercise and Brain Health: Protecting Cognition and Preventing Neurodegeneration

Exercise profoundly protects and strengthens our brains. It helps preserve cognitive abilities, sharpens mental clarity, and substantially lowers the risk of debilitating neurodegenerative diseases such as Alzheimer's, Parkinson's, and vascular dementia. Although aging naturally involves structural and functional brain changes—including memory decline, slower processing speeds, and diminished executive functions—regular physical activity powerfully counteracts these effects. By bolstering neural resilience, exercise sustains cognitive vitality throughout life.

At the heart of these protective benefits is neuroplasticity, the remarkable ability of our brains to reorganize, form new neural connections, and adapt continuously. Exercise enhances this neuroplasticity by boosting levels of brain-derived neurotrophic factor (BDNF), a critical protein that supports neuron survival, strengthens synaptic connections, and fosters the creation of new neural pathways. Elevated BDNF concentrations consistently correlate with improved memory, enhanced learning abilities, and greater cognitive flexibility, whereas lower levels accelerate cognitive decline. Aerobic activities like walking, running, and cycling excel at increasing BDNF, amplifying the brain's adaptability at every age. Remarkably, brain imaging studies consistently show that physically active people maintain a larger hippocampus—the brain region integral to memory formation and spatial navigation—underscoring the lasting structural benefits of regular movement.

Exercise further promotes brain health by enhancing cerebral blood flow (CBF). This ensures neurons continually receive essential nutrients and oxygen necessary for optimal function. As we age, vascular health tends to decline, restricting blood flow to vital cognitive regions. Regular physical activity encourages angiogenesis, the formation of new blood vessels, particularly within the hippocampus and prefrontal cortex—areas crucial for memory and executive decision-making. Improved circulation not only nourishes neurons but also facilitates efficient clearance of metabolic waste, minimizing oxidative stress and inflammation, both strongly linked to neurodegeneration. Consequently, physically active adults consistently demonstrate denser brain vasculature, greater neural efficiency, and fewer markers of cognitive decline, such as white matter lesions.

Perhaps most compellingly, regular exercise can slow or even alleviate the progression of neurodegenerative diseases. In Alzheimer's disease, characterized by harmful beta-amyloid plaques and tau tangles disrupting neuronal communication, physical activity enhances glial cell activity, supporting the brain's ability to clear these toxic proteins and slow cognitive decline. Likewise, in Parkinson's disease, where progressive loss of dopamine-producing neurons impairs motor function, exercise stimulates dopamine release, enhances motor control, and preserves neuronal function, thereby prolonging independence and mobility. Regular physical activity also reduces neuroinflammation, a shared factor in these diseases, by lowering inflammatory markers such as TNF-α and IL-6. Additionally, by improving insulin sensitivity and metabolic health, regular exercise offers further protection against cognitive decline and dementia.

Various forms of physical activity each deliver unique neurocognitive benefits. Aerobic exercises are especially potent at enhancing cerebral circulation and maintaining hippocampal integrity. Mind-body practices, including yoga and tai chi, notably reduce stress-related mental decline while promoting emotional stability. Strength training has been shown to bolster executive functioning, preserve white matter integrity, and lower dementia risk. Meanwhile, skill-based activities like dance, sports, and martial arts uniquely challenge motor coordination, reaction speed, and cognitive agility, fostering robust neural pathways and reinforcing the vital connection between brain and body.

In the final analysis, engaging regularly in exercise is an empowering commitment to lifelong cognitive resilience and adaptability. While no single activity can entirely eliminate the risk of neurodegenerative decline, consistent physical movement remains one of the most reliable and scientifically validated strategies for sustaining sharpness, clarity, and overall brain health throughout life.

The Far-Reaching Impact of Exercise on Mental and Emotional Health

Exercise does more than benefit physical health—it profoundly influences emotional well-being and psychological resilience. When the body moves, it directly influences brain chemistry, stimulating the release of neurotransmitters such as endorphins and serotonin. These biochemical messengers uplift mood, ease anxiety, and foster emotional balance. The effects of this biochemical boost are not temporary; they build over time, reinforcing long-term emotional stability, improving sleep quality, and strengthening the brain's intrinsic ability to manage stress.

Consider the constant strain that chronic stress imposes on both mental and physical health—it erodes well-being like a persistent drip wearing away stone. Exercise acts as a counterweight, helping regulate cortisol, the body's primary stress hormone. While short-term elevations in cortisol are necessary for adaptive responses, prolonged elevation can lead to anxiety, depression, and systemic inflammation. Regular movement moderates this response, cultivating a sense of calm and control. Certain practices—especially yoga and tai chi—not only fortify the body but also activate the parasympathetic nervous system, the body's innate relaxation mechanism. Thus, consistent physical activity equips people to navigate daily stressors with enhanced clarity and composure.

Beyond biochemical balance, exercise cultivates mental resilience, perseverance, and discipline—qualities that extend far beyond the physical act itself. The challenges encountered during physical activity, whether pushing through fatigue during a run, mastering a difficult yoga pose, or completing a demanding strength workout, echo the psychological endurance required in everyday life. Strength training, endurance exercise, and high-intensity interval training all engage the neural circuits responsible for overcoming adversity. By regularly activating these pathways, we sharpen our focus, heighten self-efficacy, and fortify emotional strength. Indeed, research consistently demonstrates that those participating in structured exercise programs experience greater emotional regulation, lower anxiety, and improved self-confidence, equipping them to handle life's uncertainties with greater resilience.

Exercise also supports social connection, a crucial but often overlooked component of emotional well-being. Activities such as group workouts, team sports, or even casual walks with friends create opportunities for meaningful interaction, mutual support, and shared experiences, all of which help reduce loneliness and increase life satisfaction. Research consistently demonstrates that people who participate in social exercise activities report greater emotional health and improved stress resilience compared to those who exercise alone. Even simple interactions—a friendly greeting during a morning jog or the camaraderie of a neighborhood yoga class—can lift mood and foster a deeper sense of community. Exercise delivers far more than physical fitness alone; it enhances cognitive function, promotes emotional balance, strengthens physical coordination, and reinforces the social bonds essential for overall well-being.

Momentum for Life: A Lifetime of Movement and Growth

Throughout this chapter, we've explored how exercise enhances health by synchronizing multiple biological systems. As we conclude this chapter, reflect once more on how these interconnected concepts illustrate physical activity's unique ability to foster systemic synergy, providing benefits that far exceed isolated improvements.

Among all lifestyle choices influencing both lifespan and healthspan, exercise remains unrivaled—one of the most powerful, dependable, and universally accessible interventions available. No other habit simultaneously optimizes so many biological systems or builds such formidable defenses against aging and disease. Genetics may provide the biological blueprint and medicine may intervene when problems arise, but movement proactively reshapes the trajectory of aging rather than passively responding to its inevitable effects.

Exercise is not just protective—it is a force multiplier, amplifying longevity by surpassing genetic predispositions and even outperforming many medical treatments in preventing chronic disease, preserving functional independence, and maintaining overall health. It fortifies the heart, safeguards the brain, regulates metabolism, and maintains the integrity of muscle and bone—all essential for remaining physically capable and mentally engaged as the years progress. Yet its influence penetrates deeper still. At the cellular level, exercise actively counters aging, activating repair mechanisms, enhancing mitochondrial function, and sustaining the regenerative capacity of tissues and organs. More than a health practice; it is a catalyst for continual renewal.

Even the smallest movements accumulate significant long-term benefits. A short daily walk, taking the stairs instead of the elevator, standing periodically throughout the day—these seemingly minor choices resonate across a lifetime, reinforcing resilience, adaptability, and longevity. The objective is not rigid perfection but consistent engagement, ensuring the body remains strong, flexible, and capable throughout life's many stages.

Exercise does more than extend lifespan—it fundamentally elevates the biological integrity and functional richness of the years lived. Among all longevity strategies, movement endures as the most potent, scientifically validated, and universally accessible tool available.

CHAPTER 5

Nutrition for Longevity: The Science Behind Food and Health

"Let food be thy medicine and medicine be thy food."
—HIPPOCRATES

Nutrition does more than meet one of our basic needs for survival—it is a vital force shaping longevity and overall well-being. Research continues to illuminate the intricate ways food influences human biology at every level, from the genes that regulate aging to the delicate microbial communities within the gut that support health. Beyond sustenance, thoughtful dietary choices optimize bodily functions, enhance resilience, and extend both lifespan and healthspan. While popular discussions frequently revolve around counting calories or adhering to trending diets, the deeper secret to longevity lies in grasping how specific nutrients interact harmoniously with the body's complex internal systems. As science deepens our understanding of the connection between diet and aging, nutrition remains among the most practical, accessible, and powerful tools for living a longer, healthier life.

Because nutrition has already been explored extensively—in countless books, detailed scientific studies, and abundant media coverage—this chapter intentionally adopts a lighter, more practical approach. Rather than examining complex biochemical pathways or exhaustive nutritional data, it emphasizes essential insights and foundational principles in clear, accessible language. The goal is not to replicate widely available information but to distill nutritional wisdom into actionable strategies you can readily incorporate into daily life. In essence, this chapter views nutrition as both an art and a science, blending thoughtful nuance with everyday simplicity to support your pursuit of longevity.

A Cellular Perspective: Combating Oxidative Stress and Chronic Inflammation

Aging progresses gradually and imperceptibly at the cellular level, where trillions of cells steadily accumulate damage from oxidative stress, metabolic inefficiencies, and chronic inflammation. These factors accelerate functional decline and increase disease susceptibility. Oxidative stress, characterized by an excess of free radicals, disrupts cellular health by damaging DNA, degrading proteins, and compromising cellular membranes. Dietary antioxidants provide a potent defense, neutralizing free radicals and preserving cellular integrity. Foods rich in antioxidants—such as blueberries, spinach, walnuts, vitamin C-rich citrus fruits, and vitamin E-rich nuts, seeds, and avocados—support the body's defense against oxidative damage.

Chronic inflammation also significantly contributes to aging, driving cardiovascular disease, neurodegenerative conditions, and other age-related disorders. Dietary patterns either exacerbate or reduce this persistent immune activation. Omega-3 fatty acids, abundant in fatty fish like salmon and mackerel, flaxseeds, and walnuts, function as powerful anti-inflammatory agents, modulating immune responses and protecting tissues from cumulative damage. Additionally, Coenzyme Q10, found in spinach, organ meats, and supplements, boosts mitochondrial efficiency, helping cells generate energy and reduce oxidative stress. Maintaining optimal mitochondrial function is vital for preserving cellular health, resilience, and overall wellness throughout aging.

Metabolic Balance, Caloric Restriction, and Time-Restricted Eating

Maintaining metabolic stability is essential for healthy aging. Disruptions—often caused by excessive sugar intake, inactivity, and irregular eating habits—can trigger chronic inflammation, insulin resistance, and oxidative stress, significantly increasing the risk of diabetes, cardiovascular issues, and neurodegenerative conditions like Alzheimer's and Parkinson's.

Caloric restriction (CR), defined as reducing daily calorie intake without nutritional deficits, effectively addresses these disruptions. Animal studies consistently show CR extends lifespan, sometimes by up to 40%. Although human studies have not reported equally dramatic longevity effects, they clearly demonstrate CR's positive impact on metabolic health by improving insulin sensitivity, lowering inflammation, and optimizing cholesterol levels.

Because strict caloric restriction can be difficult to maintain long-term, time-restricted eating (TRE)—limiting food intake to a specific daily window (such as 8–12 hours)—provides a practical alternative with similar metabolic advantages. TRE effectively improves insulin sensitivity and reduces inflammation without requiring significant calorie reductions.

Additionally, nutrient-rich and polyphenol-rich foods like green tea, dark chocolate, and berries amplify these effects by activating autophagy, a vital cellular housekeeping process. Autophagy removes damaged proteins, dysfunctional organelles, and accumulated metabolic waste, enhancing cellular function and promoting longevity.

Together, caloric restriction, time-restricted eating, and targeted nutritional choices form a powerful framework for restoring metabolic equilibrium, reducing disease risk, and supporting lasting physical and cognitive function. Chapter 7 provides comprehensive guidance on these dietary strategies, including detailed mechanisms and practical implementation advice.

The Gut Microbiome: Nutrition's Silent Partner

Hidden deep within the digestive tract exists a dynamic community of trillions of microorganisms, quietly contributing to overall wellness and longevity. Known collectively as the gut microbiome, this expansive microbial network actively facilitates digestion, fortifies immunity, and even influences mental and emotional well-being. Central to nurturing this ecosystem is dietary fiber, which serves as essential nourishment for beneficial bacteria. Fiber-rich foods—including beans simmered into hearty soups, oats stirred into comforting porridge, leafy greens tossed in crisp salads, and whole grains baked into wholesome breads—contain prebiotics. These specialized fibers stimulate the growth and resilience of favorable microbes, maintaining microbial diversity vital for optimal digestive function.

Complementing dietary fiber, probiotics—live beneficial microorganisms found naturally in fermented foods—further enhance microbial health. Consuming fermented products such as tangy yogurt, kefir smoothies, spicy kimchi, crisp sauerkraut, and savory miso soups helps sustain a balanced and flourishing gut environment. Research increasingly links regular probiotic intake with improved digestive comfort, reduced inflammation, and enhanced cognitive function, highlighting the importance of the gut-brain axis, a communication pathway connecting the intestines with the central nervous system.

However, certain dietary habits may compromise this balance. Regular consumption of processed foods, refined carbohydrates, and artificial sweeteners can encourage harmful bacterial growth, potentially leading to dysbiosis—a disrupted microbial state associated with chronic inflammation, insulin resistance, and metabolic dysfunction. By consciously emphasizing fiber-rich, whole-food ingredients and minimizing intake of ultra-processed options, the gut microbiome remains a reliable partner in maintaining metabolic health and reinforcing the body's natural defenses.

The Mediterranean Diet: A Model for Longevity

Among the many dietary patterns studied for longevity, the Mediterranean diet stands apart as one of the most extensively researched and consistently effective for enhancing both healthspan and lifespan. Rooted deeply in the traditional eating habits of Mediterranean regions, this approach embraces whole, minimally processed foods—abundant fresh fruits, fresh vegetables, nourishing whole grains, crunchy nuts, wholesome seeds, and rich extra virgin olive oil. It also incorporates moderate amounts of fish, poultry, and dairy products as sources of high-quality protein, while red meat and processed foods are enjoyed sparingly. Rather than rigid rules or restrictive meal plans, this diet celebrates flavorful, nutrient-dense ingredients that sustain cellular health and protect the body from chronic diseases.

The cardiovascular benefits of the Mediterranean diet are particularly remarkable. The landmark PREDIMED Study (2013)—a large-scale, randomized trial conducted in Spain—revealed a striking 30% reduction in major cardiovascular events, including heart attack, stroke, and cardiovascular-related death, among participants following a Mediterranean diet supplemented with extra virgin olive oil or nuts, compared to those adhering to a low-fat diet. These findings were further supported by a 2019 meta-analysis of multiple cohort studies, which confirmed that strong adherence to this diet lowered cardiovascular mortality risk by 25%. By effectively reducing inflammation, enhancing circulation, and supporting healthier lipid profiles, this dietary pattern provides significant protection against heart disease.

Beyond cardiovascular health, the Mediterranean diet plays a significant role in longevity. Observational studies from Blue Zones—regions globally recognized for their high concentrations of people enjoying exceptional health and extended lifespans—demonstrate the life-prolonging power of Mediterranean-style eating. Consider the residents of Sardinia, Italy, whose traditional meals center around legumes simmered in stews, whole grains in rustic breads, and healthy fats like olive oil drizzled generously over fresh vegetables—staples of the Mediterranean diet.

A 2014 meta-analysis published in the *British Journal of Nutrition*, titled "Mediterranean diet and its components in relation to all-cause mortality," integrated findings from multiple studies to assess the diet's impact on lifespan. The results consistently demonstrated that greater adherence to Mediterranean dietary patterns was associated with lower all-cause mortality, positioning this eating style as a compelling dietary framework for enhancing both the duration and quality of life.

Cognitive health, too, receives substantial protection from the Mediterranean diet. A 2021 study published in *Neurology* showed that people closely following this diet experienced slower cognitive decline and a significantly lower risk of Alzheimer's disease. This protective effect arises from the diet's plentiful omega-3 fatty acids, polyphenols, and antioxidants, compounds that combat neuroinflammation and oxidative stress while preserving neuronal function. Furthermore, the MIND diet—a thoughtful hybrid combining the Mediterranean diet and the DASH diet (a nutritional approach designed to lower blood pressure)—demonstrated remarkable efficacy, reducing Alzheimer's risk by up to 53% in those who consistently adhered to its guidelines.

Metabolic health also flourishes within the context of this dietary approach. A notable study published in *Diabetes Care* found that the Mediterranean diet enhances insulin sensitivity and stabilizes blood sugar levels, largely owing to its focus on fiber-rich foods, healthy fats, and balanced carbohydrates. Further supporting these findings, a 2019 review confirmed its effectiveness in weight management, showing that adherence to the Mediterranean diet promotes sustained weight loss and long-term metabolic well-being. Thus, it serves as a practical, flexible, and effective approach for preventing type 2 diabetes.

Cancer prevention is another compelling advantage of the Mediterranean diet. Its abundance of antioxidants and anti-inflammatory compounds—such as polyphenols in olive oil and flavonoids in colorful fruits and vegetables—helps neutralize oxidative stress and suppress chronic inflammation, both critical drivers of cancer development.

Reinforcing these findings, a 2020 meta-analysis published in *Nutrition Reviews* reported that people with high adherence to the Mediterranean diet exhibited significantly lower risks of colorectal, breast, and gastric cancers, further solidifying its protective role against malignancies.

What makes the Mediterranean diet uniquely effective is its synergistic blend of nutrients and bioactive compounds. Rich in antioxidants and polyphenols, it protects cells from oxidative damage and DNA mutations. Its anti-inflammatory effects, derived largely from ingredients like olive oil, nuts, and fatty fish, counteract chronic inflammation, a major driver of aging and disease. Moreover, the diet's fiber-rich foundation nourishes the gut microbiome, bolstering digestive health, immune function, and overall systemic well-being. Its balanced macronutrient profile—high in healthy fats, moderate in protein, and rich in complex carbohydrates—optimizes energy regulation and metabolic efficiency, reinforcing its well-deserved reputation as one of the most effective dietary strategies for maintaining metabolic integrity and delaying age-related decline.

The Power of Energy Balance: Understanding Calories In vs. Calories Out

Trendy diets like keto, Mediterranean, and intermittent fasting often dominate popular discussions around weight loss and health. Yet beneath all these varied strategies lies a foundational principle that remains constant: energy balance—the fundamental relationship between calories consumed and calories expended—ultimately governs weight management and metabolic health. The underlying equation is elegantly simple: when calorie intake exceeds energy expenditure, the body stores the surplus as fat. Conversely, when expenditure surpasses intake, stored energy reserves are tapped, facilitating fat loss.

However, energy balance shapes far more than just body weight. It significantly influences metabolic function, hormonal regulation, and disease prevention. Maintaining a healthy weight enhances insulin sensitivity, reduces systemic inflammation, and significantly lowers the risk of chronic conditions such as type 2 diabetes and heart disease. While the nutritional quality of food remains crucial for overall health, understanding how energy intake aligns thoughtfully with expenditure forms the bedrock of sustainable weight control.

This framework also offers remarkable flexibility. Whether a person follows a plant-based diet, a low-carbohydrate approach, or a personalized hybrid pattern tailored to their preferences, energy balance accommodates diverse dietary styles. Instead of chasing fleeting dietary trends, mastering the core principles of energy dynamics fosters a more sustainable and adaptable pathway to lasting health.

More fundamentally, embracing energy balance represents awareness rather than restriction. It is not a rigid dogma but rather a guiding principle that encourages informed, mindful decisions around food and physical activity. By understanding clearly how the body regulates energy, one can confidently navigate nutritional choices, maintain metabolic flexibility, and sustain lifelong well-being without unnecessary complexity.

Nourishing a Long and Healthy Life

Nutrition is far more than basic sustenance. It serves as a cornerstone of longevity, intricately influencing cellular vitality, immune resilience, and metabolic efficiency. Every dietary choice we make today shapes both immediate wellness and long-term health outcomes. At a fundamental level, nutrients modulate essential biological pathways that regulate metabolism, inflammation, and cellular regeneration—processes critical to our bodies' ability to handle stress, maintain internal balance, and preserve physical and cognitive function as we age.

Thoughtfully selected foods become active partners in sustaining health. Antioxidant-rich fruits, such as blueberries, and leafy greens like kale combat oxidative stress. Whole grains—quinoa, oats, and barley—enhance digestive efficiency and metabolic stability. Beneficial fats from avocados and olive oil support cardiovascular health and strengthen cellular membranes, while essential micronutrients from nuts and seeds enhance systemic resilience. Collectively, these dietary choices help manage inflammation, lower chronic disease risk, and sustain cognitive sharpness. Clearly, wise nutritional habits enhance physical capability, mental clarity, and emotional well-being throughout life.

Nutrition also extends beyond biology. It embodies cultural heritage, personal identity, and emotional connections. Recipes passed down through generations, carefully prepared meals, and meaningful food rituals enrich community ties and individual identity. How do we reconcile scientific guidance with cherished culinary traditions? By thoughtfully blending nutritional science with meaningful practices, we create a sustainable pathway to long-term health. In this way, family gatherings can center around dishes that preserve cultural meaning while incorporating nutritional insights, simultaneously supporting physical well-being and enriching social bonds.

Pursuing nutritional longevity isn't about rigid dietary perfection. Instead, it thrives on consistent, intentional choices that respect individual differences, preferences, and lifestyles. Embracing flexibility, moderation, and enjoyment ensures nutritional practices remain sustainable and effective over time.

Every nutritional choice resonates deeply within our cells, shaping the story of our resilience, mental agility, and autonomy in later years. By consciously blending the precision of nutritional science with the richness of culinary tradition, we nourish not only longevity but a life anchored in cherished relationships, cultural identity, and shared experiences.

CHAPTER 6

Beyond Diet—Supplements and Functional Foods That Work

"Knowledge is the food of the soul."
—PLATO

Dietary supplements and functional foods occupy a distinct niche in the broader ecosystem of longevity. They're neither miracle cures nor simply nutritional extras; instead, think of them as specialized species within a complex biological community—each uniquely adapted to support and enhance a foundational diet and lifestyle. While nourishing food remains the bedrock of healthy aging, targeted supplements can help address important challenges that emerge over time, including chronic inflammation, oxidative stress, declining mitochondrial efficiency, accumulating senescent cells, and diminished autophagy—the body's intrinsic cellular maintenance process.

But supplements aren't equally beneficial for everyone. Genetics, diet quality, lifestyle habits, and current health status all influence how effectively a supplement will perform. Supplements can't replace a healthy lifestyle; instead, they complement and enhance it. Imagine health as a carefully designed home: nutritious food, regular exercise, quality sleep, and effective stress management form the foundation, walls, and framework.

Supplements, then, are like the fine details and carefully chosen finishes—important enhancements that elevate and complete the structure, but meaningful only if the core design is sound. Given the wide array of options available, this chapter emphasizes supplements and foods with robust scientific backing, focusing on those most likely to genuinely support healthy aging.

How Supplements Fit into the Aging Equation

Supplements function by providing targeted support—addressing specific nutritional shortfalls or bolstering biological processes that naturally become less efficient with age. Consider omega-3 supplements, which reinforce the body's resilience against inflammation and cognitive decline, or vitamin D, which directs calcium to bones precisely where it's needed. However, it's essential to keep expectations realistic: supplements rarely produce immediate, dramatic effects. Instead, their true value emerges gradually, enhancing the body's existing systems when combined with the nutrients naturally found in whole foods.

Eating antioxidant-rich foods like berries, greens, or nuts provides a spectrum of nutrients that supplements alone typically can't replicate. Even so, strategic supplementation can amplify these natural effects. For instance, a diet rich in polyphenols paired with targeted antioxidants might provide enhanced cellular protection beyond diet alone. Yet, this synergy also highlights a critical caveat: isolated supplements sometimes fail to deliver benefits seen in whole foods, and impressive results from laboratory studies often translate into smaller, less consistent outcomes in humans.

In the final analysis, supplements are most effective when thoughtfully integrated into a broader lifestyle strategy—one grounded firmly in balanced nutrition, consistent exercise, restful sleep, and healthy stress management. Approached in this comprehensive manner, supplements can become meaningful allies in the pursuit of sustained health and vitality throughout the aging process.

Omega-3s and Vitamin D: Building Blocks for a Sharper Brain and Stronger Bones

Omega-3 fatty acids—particularly EPA, abundant in foods like salmon, flaxseeds, and walnuts—do much more than protect the heart. Think of omega-3s as high-quality fuel that helps keep the brain performing smoothly. Research consistently shows that people who regularly consume omega-3-rich foods or supplements experience clearer thinking, sharper memory, and a slower pace of cognitive aging. There's even early evidence hinting at reduced risks for neurodegenerative conditions like Alzheimer's disease—though definitive proof is still forthcoming. If regularly eating fish isn't practical, supplements can offer a reliable alternative.

Vitamin D, another essential nutrient, acts a bit like a supervisor directing calcium exactly where it's needed most—bones. Yet many educated adults, especially those in northern climates or who spend limited time outdoors, unknowingly live with chronic vitamin D deficiency. Over time, this shortfall contributes to weaker bones, greater fracture risk, and diminished immunity. Interestingly, combining vitamin D3 with vitamin K2 might amplify its effectiveness, helping calcium find its way precisely into bone structure, rather than accumulating where it could cause trouble, such as in arteries. Although the science around ideal dosages and long-term benefits is still evolving, this nutrient pairing offers a practical approach for those prioritizing skeletal and cardiovascular health into later life.

Creatine: Reimagining an Athletic Supplement for Healthy Aging

Creatine might evoke images of bodybuilders and competitive athletes, but it's increasingly clear this compound offers meaningful advantages beyond sports performance. With age, significant changes occur over time—a bit less muscle strength, somewhat slower recovery, perhaps diminished confidence in your physical balance. Creatine acts like a cellular energy reserve, giving muscles the boost they need to stay stronger and perform more reliably, reducing everyday risks like falls or impaired mobility.

More intriguingly, recent studies suggest creatine might also support cognitive agility, particularly enhancing memory and reaction speed in older adults who've started to notice age-related cognitive slowing. While these improvements are typically modest—not transformative miracles—they can still translate into tangible benefits in everyday life, like quicker recall and sharper focus. Given creatine's safety, affordability, and convenience, it represents a realistic addition to a longevity-focused lifestyle.

CoQ10 and NAD+: Supporting Cellular Energy for Sustained Vitality

With age, it may feel as though one's internal batteries no longer hold their charge as reliably as they once did. Behind this common sense of fatigue and reduced stamina lies a biological reality: the mitochondria, tiny cellular power plants responsible for energy production, become less efficient over time. Coenzyme Q10 (CoQ10) plays a crucial role in keeping these power plants running smoothly. Levels of CoQ10 naturally decline as you get older, and medications like statins (used to control cholesterol) further lower them. Supplementing with CoQ10 can help restore this energy balance, potentially improving daily vitality and cardiovascular function.

In parallel, NAD+ is emerging as another critical player. Think of NAD+ as the conductor in the orchestra of cellular health, essential for keeping metabolism in tune and DNA repair mechanisms active. NAD+ levels drop gradually as you age, possibly accelerating aspects of cellular aging. Compounds like NMN and NR, which can boost NAD+ within cells, have shown promising initial results in improving metabolic health and mitochondrial efficiency in early human trials. But it's important to remain realistic—the science is still young. Questions remain about optimal doses, long-term safety, and exactly how significant their real-world impact will be. Given their potential importance, NAD+, NMN, and NR receive more detailed attention in a later chapter, where the latest research and practical considerations are explored thoroughly.

Antioxidants and Aging: Resveratrol, Polyphenols & Curcumin

Resveratrol, the compound famously linked to red wine, grapes, and berries, often garners attention in longevity discussions. However, consuming a glass or two of red wine does not meaningfully enhance resveratrol intake—the amounts naturally present in foods are simply too small. Instead, supplements provide higher concentrations, potentially sufficient to influence key pathways associated with aging. In laboratory studies, resveratrol activates proteins known as sirtuins, which help cells manage stress, reduce inflammation, and support DNA repair. Although these findings appear promising, translating them directly into human benefits has proven challenging, with results varying significantly between studies. Nevertheless, certain markers of metabolic health and inflammation do show improvement, suggesting some practical value.

Polyphenols—a large family of antioxidants abundant in foods such as blueberries, olive oil, and dark chocolate—might best be thought of as small daily investments rather than dramatic interventions. Regularly eating polyphenol-rich foods appears to moderate inflammation and oxidative damage, somewhat akin to consistent, modest exercise. Though their impact may not be dramatic or immediate, sustained habits accumulate gradually over time, potentially protecting cardiovascular function and preserving cognitive health.

Curcumin, turmeric's bright yellow active ingredient, has gained popularity largely due to its anti-inflammatory properties. When turmeric is recommended for joint pain, curcumin is typically the reason. Clinical studies indicate that curcumin supplements can moderately ease discomfort and inflammation, particularly in cases involving conditions such as osteoarthritis. However, a practical challenge remains: curcumin is notoriously difficult for the body to absorb. To address this limitation, supplements commonly pair curcumin with ingredients like black pepper extract (piperine), significantly enhancing absorption and effectiveness.

Clearing Senescent Cells: Fisetin and Quercetin

Senescent cells are like worn-out machinery that, instead of quietly breaking down and being recycled, linger and clutter up the workspace. Over time, these dysfunctional cells accumulate, releasing inflammatory signals that negatively affect tissues and contribute to aging-related decline. To address this, scientists have explored natural plant compounds known as flavonoids—specifically fisetin (found in strawberries) and quercetin (abundant in apples and onions). Animal studies suggest these compounds can selectively eliminate senescent cells, potentially reducing inflammation and improving tissue function.

While human studies on these senolytics are still in their infancy, early results show promise. It's important, however, to recognize that these findings aren't yet definitive. Larger, rigorous studies are needed to determine effective dosages, clarify long-term safety, and confirm their actual impact on human aging. Despite this, the underlying science is compelling enough to justify cautious optimism.

Cellular Housekeeping with Spermidine

Autophagy—the cells' internal recycling process—is crucial but often overlooked. Think of autophagy as routine housekeeping, essential to keeping cells tidy and functional. With age, cells become less efficient at this cleanup, leading to a buildup of damaged materials, somewhat like clutter accumulating in a neglected room. Spermidine, naturally found in wheat germ, soybeans, and aged cheese, appears to stimulate this housekeeping process, helping cells stay healthier longer.

People who eat diets naturally richer in spermidine tend to have better cardiovascular health and even slightly longer lifespans, at least according to observational studies. Early human trials suggest potential cognitive and anti-inflammatory benefits as well, though it's still too early to draw definitive conclusions. Further research is essential to confirm these promising indications, define the most effective doses, and establish long-term safety. Nonetheless, given its safety profile and presence in common foods, including spermidine-rich items in one's diet may be a practical strategy for supporting healthy aging.

Gut Health: Probiotics, Prebiotics & Fermented Foods in Longevity

The gut microbiome influences far more than digestion alone; it shapes immunity, metabolic stability, and even cognitive health. With age, microbial diversity in the gut often diminishes, potentially leading to increased inflammation and reduced resilience to illness. Regularly incorporating fermented foods—like yogurt, kefir, kimchi, or sauerkraut—can help restore beneficial bacterial communities and modulate inflammatory responses. Probiotics in these foods don't just replenish bacteria; studies indicate they encourage microbial diversity linked with healthier aging.

But probiotic bacteria need sustenance. Prebiotics, fibers from foods like onions, ripe bananas, garlic, and whole grains, provide nourishment for beneficial microbes. Prebiotics might be thought of as the rich, nutrient-dense soil where beneficial bacteria flourish. This balanced microbial environment supports not only gut function but systemic health, particularly important as the body navigates the stresses of aging.

Fiber Supplements: Supporting Gut and Metabolic Health

Ideally, fiber would come primarily from diet—plenty of vegetables, legumes, fruits, and whole grains. However, dietary habits and appetite often change with age, making adequate fiber intake more challenging. Fiber supplements like psyllium husk or inulin can effectively bridge this gap. Clinical trials consistently demonstrate psyllium's ability to significantly reduce LDL cholesterol and regulate blood sugar, essential for long-term cardiovascular health. Likewise, inulin specifically nourishes beneficial gut bacteria, helping to maintain a stable and diverse microbiome. Although supplements shouldn't replace dietary fiber entirely, they're practical tools when dietary fiber intake falls short.

Collagen Peptides & Magnesium: Structural Support for Aging

Collagen provides structural integrity to skin, joints, and bones. Yet natural collagen synthesis diminishes gradually as we age, contributing to wrinkles, reduced joint mobility, and weaker connective tissue. Recent clinical studies have reported modest improvements in skin hydration, elasticity, and joint comfort with consistent collagen peptide supplementation. Results aren't dramatic for everyone, but many people do notice meaningful benefits.

Similarly, magnesium is critical for numerous bodily functions, from muscle contraction and nerve signaling to glucose metabolism and bone density. Despite its importance, magnesium deficiency is common, especially among older adults, elevating the risk for cardiovascular issues (including arrhythmias such as atrial fibrillation), diabetes, and osteoporosis. While dietary sources like leafy greens, almonds, and seeds should be prioritized, supplemental magnesium can safely help maintain adequate levels if dietary intake is insufficient.

Green Tea and EGCG: Everyday Support for Metabolism and Health

Green tea has moved beyond tradition into serious scientific exploration. Its best-known compound, EGCG, acts like a prodding persistent defense system—helping the body manage inflammation and support metabolic health. Populations that drink green tea regularly, particularly in parts of Asia, often experience lower rates of heart disease, cognitive decline, and some cancers. Controlled human studies back this up, showing modest but measurable improvements in blood sugar regulation, cholesterol levels, and weight management.

However, moderation is key. Just as concentrating sunlight through a magnifying glass can create unintended heat, extracting EGCG into high-dose supplements can occasionally pose risks, such as liver problems. The sensible approach is to enjoy green tea as a beverage or to use moderate-dose extracts, safely benefiting from its supportive effects without pushing the body beyond healthy limits.

Whole Grains, Nuts, and Seeds: Building Blocks for Metabolic Stability

Whole grains—such as oats, barley, and quinoa—are nutritional slow burners. Unlike refined grains, which cause rapid blood sugar spikes, these complex carbohydrates provide sustained, steady energy. They also feed beneficial gut bacteria, offering indirect yet meaningful support for overall health. A simple but effective practice—like swapping refined breakfast cereals for hearty oats or choosing whole-grain bread instead of white bread—can make a significant difference over years, stabilizing metabolism and improving cardiovascular health.

Similarly, nuts and seeds like almonds, walnuts, flax, and chia are nutritional powerhouses packaged neatly by nature. Just a small handful daily provides omega-3 fatty acids, antioxidants, and fiber, which help reduce inflammation, support heart health, and even sharpen cognitive performance. While nuts and seeds won't instantly transform one's health, think of their impact as small, consistent deposits in a wellness account—gradually accumulating value over time.

Multivitamins: Filling the Nutritional Gaps

Even those dedicated to healthy eating can encounter nutritional shortfalls—particularly as age affects how efficiently nutrients are absorbed or utilized. Nutrients like vitamin B12, zinc, and magnesium are common examples. Clinical studies consistently show modest cognitive improvements and better overall nutrient status among older adults regularly taking a multivitamin.

Still, no supplement can fully replicate the complexity of real food. Think of a multivitamin as nutritional insurance: not designed to replace a balanced diet, but valuable in ensuring consistent nutritional coverage, particularly during times when dietary variety becomes limited.

A Thoughtful Approach to Nutrition and Longevity

Supplements and functional foods aren't shortcuts or miracle solutions. Instead, consider them specialized tools—fine-tuned additions that can enhance a foundation you've already established through good habits. Ingredients like creatine, spermidine, fiber supplements, and green tea extracts don't magically reverse aging. Rather, they support crucial processes—reducing chronic inflammation, protecting against oxidative stress, enhancing mitochondrial function, and improving the cellular "housekeeping" process of autophagy.

Nevertheless, more isn't always better. Excessive or careless supplementation can sometimes backfire—for example, high-dose antioxidants might disrupt the body's natural ability to adapt to mild stresses, a process crucial for cellular resilience. Precision and personalization matter. Advances in genetics, biomarker testing, and personalized health assessments may allow supplementation strategies to become more targeted and effective, aligning closely with an individual's physiology.

In the end, optimal health and longevity result from integrating dietary supplements thoughtfully within a comprehensive lifestyle strategy. Nutrient-rich whole foods, regular physical activity, quality sleep, and proactive stress management remain the most important pillars. Together, these practices and targeted supplementation help maintain mental clarity, physical strength, and overall vitality—allowing people to experience healthy aging not just theoretically, but practically, in daily life.

CHAPTER 7

Fasting and Caloric Restriction: Activating Cellular Renewal

"To lengthen thy life, lessen thy meals."
—BENJAMIN FRANKLIN

Could the secret to a longer, healthier life lie not just in the foods we consume, but also in when and how much we eat? Throughout most of human history, fasting wasn't only a lifestyle choice—it was a necessity, dictated by the ebb and flow of available resources. These cycles of feast and famine shaped our metabolism, refining the body's innate ability to endure scarcity and thrive despite hardship. Modern abundance, however, has largely erased these natural fasting periods, potentially accelerating aging and increasing vulnerability to chronic diseases. Yet emerging research reveals that deliberately reintroducing these ancestral eating patterns through caloric restriction and intermittent fasting may offer an effective approach to restoring metabolic balance, revitalizing cellular health, and possibly even extending lifespan.

Far from mere weight-loss fads, these dietary practices tap into deeply conserved biological mechanisms evolved over millennia. They enhance energy metabolism, regulate hormonal balance, reduce inflammation, and activate the body's sophisticated cellular repair processes. Unlike conventional diets, which typically emphasize short-term aesthetic goals, caloric restriction and intermittent fasting operate at a fundamental, molecular level, slowing down critical processes implicated in aging and chronic disease.

Caloric Restriction: A Controlled Approach to Longevity

Caloric restriction (CR) represents much more than simply cutting back on food—it is a carefully calibrated practice of reducing energy intake while preserving essential nutrition. For nearly a century, scientists have studied CR's profound impacts, particularly in animal models. Remarkably, reducing caloric intake by 20 to 40 percent consistently extends lifespan and delays age-associated diseases in laboratory settings. Although human longevity outcomes are still under rigorous exploration, compelling evidence from studies like the groundbreaking CALERIE trial (Comprehensive Assessment of Long-term Effects of Reducing Intake of Energy)—a rigorous, controlled study examining moderate caloric restriction in healthy, non-obese adults—indicates that even modest calorie reduction significantly reduces inflammation, strengthens cardiovascular health, enhances insulin sensitivity, and optimizes metabolic function.

On a cellular level, caloric restriction triggers a shift toward enhanced metabolic efficiency. The body responds to this mild nutritional stress by conserving energy, repairing accumulated cellular damage, and allocating resources strategically for maintenance rather than growth. A vital element of this adaptive response is autophagy, the body's inherent recycling system that diligently clears damaged and dysfunctional cellular components before they contribute to aging. Imagine autophagy as a meticulous gardener pruning away wilted leaves, ensuring a healthier, more vibrant biological environment. Additionally, CR bolsters mitochondrial function, empowering cells to effectively neutralize oxidative stress—a significant factor driving cellular degeneration. The outcome is a finely balanced, rejuvenated cellular state primed for survival and long-term resilience.

Beyond cellular renewal, CR exerts powerful hormonal effects. It modulates insulin-like growth factor-1 (IGF-1), a protein associated with growth and cell proliferation, yet also linked to aging and cancer risk. Animal studies have connected lower IGF-1 levels with increased lifespan, suggesting a biological shift from growth toward preservation and repair. However, the human relationship to IGF-1 is more nuanced. While moderate reductions may indeed support longevity, excessively low levels in aging adults correlate with muscle loss and frailty, underscoring the delicate balance necessary when fine-tuning these pathways for optimal health.

Another critical player in this process is the sirtuin family of proteins—cellular "longevity genes" responsible for orchestrating DNA repair, mitochondrial efficiency, and stress resistance. Caloric restriction activates sirtuins, enhancing the body's capacity to adapt to metabolic stresses and mitigate age-related damage. Collectively, these effects help delay the onset of age-associated diseases, underscoring that caloric restriction is not only a dietary adjustment but a fundamental biological shift toward sustained longevity and health.

Through this intricate synergy of cellular maintenance, hormonal recalibration, and metabolic optimization, caloric restriction emerges as a powerful strategy for enhancing healthspan and delaying physiological decline. Although its precise impact on human lifespan extension continues to be explored, the well-established health improvements observed in studies like CALERIE demonstrate its potential to transform how we approach aging. Caloric restriction exemplifies how strategic nutritional interventions can recalibrate our biological clock, enhancing physical and cognitive function beyond what is typically observed with aging.

Intermittent Fasting: The Power of Meal Timing

Intermittent fasting (IF) is less about restricting calories and more about strategically timing meals. Rather than focusing solely on what is eaten, IF emphasizes when food is consumed, aligning with the body's inherent capacity to seamlessly transition between energy sources. Unlike continuous caloric restriction, intermittent fasting alternates between periods of eating and fasting, prompting distinct and beneficial physiological responses during each cycle.

Various IF methods accommodate diverse lifestyles and levels of dedication. For example, the popular 16:8 protocol confines daily eating to an eight-hour window, followed by a restorative 16-hour fasting period—perhaps skipping breakfast and savoring nutritious meals between noon and early evening. The flexible 5:2 plan permits normal eating habits five days per week, while dramatically reducing calorie intake on two non-consecutive days. For individuals seeking deeper metabolic benefits, periodic fasts of 24 to 72 hours are practiced, increasingly tapping into fat oxidation and cellular rejuvenation processes.

During fasting periods, the body undergoes a remarkable metabolic transition. As glycogen stores in muscles and liver are gradually depleted, the body shifts from glucose-based metabolism toward fat oxidation, steadily producing ketones. Ketones provide a clean, efficient alternative fuel source—particularly nourishing the brain—and may help reduce oxidative stress over extended fasting durations. This adaptive shift improves insulin sensitivity, stabilizes blood sugar levels, and substantially reduces risks of type 2 diabetes and metabolic dysfunction.

Beyond metabolic shifts, intermittent fasting, like caloric restriction, activates autophagy, the cell's internal housekeeping mechanism. With reduced energy intake, cells initiate self-renewal by identifying and dismantling damaged proteins, malfunctioning organelles, and accumulated cellular debris. This cellular renewal process rejuvenates cell function and slows age-related deterioration. Autophagy's protective effects are particularly significant against neurodegenerative diseases such as Alzheimer's and Parkinson's, where accumulated misfolded proteins profoundly impact disease progression.

Intermittent fasting's benefits extend far beyond metabolism and cellular renewal—it also powerfully influences brain health. Research demonstrates that fasting boosts levels of brain-derived neurotrophic factor (BDNF), an essential protein that promotes neuronal growth, cognitive function, and neuroprotection. Elevated BDNF has been associated with improved learning and memory, suggesting IF could provide enduring neurological benefits.

Moreover, intermittent fasting has consistently demonstrated reductions in inflammatory markers, potentially decreasing risks for chronic diseases such as cardiovascular disease, cancer, and autoimmune disorders. Nevertheless, the magnitude of these benefits depends significantly upon fasting duration, individual metabolic health, and overall dietary quality. IF yields the most substantial results when thoughtfully combined with nutrient-rich eating and a balanced, health-supporting lifestyle.

Incorporating structured fasting periods allows us to engage the body's innate ability to reset, repair, and renew. More than a dietary technique, intermittent fasting reconnects us with ancient metabolic rhythms, underscoring that timing our nourishment thoughtfully might be just as essential as the nourishment itself.

How CR and IF Influence Longevity

Both caloric restriction (CR) and intermittent fasting (IF) engage deeply conserved longevity pathways, optimizing metabolic efficiency, cellular resilience, and stress adaptation. Rather than maintaining a continuous energy surplus, these dietary strategies nudge the body toward a state of carefully managed resource utilization. By lowering insulin levels, enhancing mitochondrial function, and periodically challenging metabolic pathways, CR and IF effectively reprogram cellular priorities—reinforcing the principle that periodic nutritional stress fortifies long-term health and vitality.

One hallmark metabolic adaptation triggered by prolonged fasting is ketogenesis. When glycogen stores run low, the body shifts into producing ketones as an alternative energy source—like a well-designed hybrid engine smoothly transitioning between fuel types. Ketones are far more than an emergency fuel; they act as molecular messengers, intricately regulating inflammation and oxidative stress by activating protective pathways such as

Nrf2 (a cellular protein that triggers antioxidant defenses and detoxification processes) and simultaneously inhibiting harmful mechanisms like the NLRP3 inflammasome (a protein complex involved in initiating inflammation linked to aging and chronic disease). Nevertheless, the longevity-promoting effects of caloric restriction (CR) and intermittent fasting (IF) extend well beyond ketone metabolism alone. Even without entering deep ketosis, these dietary strategies activate critical cellular repair mechanisms, enhance mitochondrial efficiency, and finely tune metabolic flexibility. Each of these processes represents a cornerstone of sustained health and extended longevity.

At the genetic level, CR and IF recalibrate the body's longevity blueprint, enhancing the activity of critical cellular regulators such as sirtuins, AMPK signaling, and insulin-like growth factor-1 (IGF-1). Sirtuins, often described as "longevity genes," orchestrate essential processes such as DNA repair, mitochondrial efficiency (the capacity of cells to efficiently produce energy while minimizing cellular stress), and cellular resilience against damage.

AMPK, the master regulator of cellular energy, shifts the body's metabolic gears from storage mode to energy optimization, promoting fat oxidation and improved glucose metabolism. Meanwhile, IGF-1, a hormone intricately linked to growth and aging, presents a fascinating paradox. Animal studies clearly link lower IGF-1 levels to increased lifespan; yet, in humans, excessive suppression could inadvertently lead to frailty, muscle loss, and weakened immune defenses. CR and IF thoughtfully modulate IGF-1, delicately balancing cellular repair mechanisms with the essential maintenance of physiological functions—much like skillfully adjusting a sail to harness the perfect wind for smooth, efficient navigation.

Another crucial longevity pathway influenced by CR and IF involves the mechanistic target of rapamycin (mTOR), a central regulator overseeing cell growth, protein synthesis, and aging. Suppressing mTOR shifts cellular priorities away from relentless growth and proliferation, instead promoting critical processes like autophagy, cellular repair, and stress resilience—patterns consistently observed in some of nature's longest-lived organisms. Yet, careful moderation is essential; excessive inhibition of mTOR can impair immune function, diminish muscle maintenance, and slow wound healing. CR and IF strategically regulate mTOR activity in a cyclical fashion, allowing growth when nutrients are plentiful and prioritizing repair during fasting or caloric restriction periods. This dynamic rhythm, a harmonious interplay between growth and renewal, underlies sustained metabolic flexibility and ultimately longevity.

By simultaneously engaging multiple interwoven longevity pathways, CR and IF foster an internal cellular environment uniquely resistant to age-related deterioration. Their true value extends well beyond lifespan extension—they also enhance healthspan, the number of vibrant, fulfilling years lived in optimal physical and cognitive condition. A longer life, after all, is most meaningful when accompanied by strength, resilience, and vitality. By incorporating strategic periods of metabolic challenge, CR and IF activate the body's innate capacity for renewal and repair, making increased longevity an achievable reality rather than a distant ideal.

Current Research on CR and IF: What We Know So Far

Animal research has provided compelling insights into the longevity-enhancing effects of caloric restriction (CR) and intermittent fasting (IF). In rodents, CR reliably extends lifespan by an impressive 20 to 50 percent, simultaneously delaying age-related diseases such as cancer, cardiovascular dysfunction, and neurodegeneration. In primate studies, CR consistently enhances healthspan, metabolic regulation, and inflammatory markers, although its exact impact on lifespan varies among studies. Intermittent fasting, while not as directly linked to longevity extension, has demonstrated remarkable benefits—boosting metabolic flexibility, fortifying cellular defenses, and protecting cognitive function across diverse species. These findings suggest that intermittent periods of energy restriction tap into ancient survival mechanisms, reinforcing cellular resilience and fostering longevity.

In human studies, directly measuring lifespan extension presents substantial challenges; nevertheless, the capacity of CR and IF to meaningfully extend healthspan—the span of life spent in optimal health—is robustly supported. For instance, the CALERIE trial revealed that even a moderate 25 percent reduction in calorie intake over two years led to significantly lower inflammation, enhanced cardiovascular function, and improved metabolic efficiency. Similarly, clinical studies on intermittent fasting offer encouraging evidence of metabolic benefits, including heightened insulin sensitivity, improved lipid profiles, and stronger markers of cognitive resilience. However, while short-term benefits are compelling, ongoing research continues to explore the long-term implications of IF on human healthspan.

Both CR and IF notably enhance metabolic flexibility—the body's elegant ability to transition seamlessly between glucose and fat metabolism based on energy availability. This optimization in fuel usage supports cellular maintenance, mitigates oxidative stress, and finely tunes energy utilization. While more research is necessary to determine whether these interventions can significantly extend human lifespan, their capacity to delay disease onset, strengthen metabolic health, and counteract age-related decline is already well documented, underscoring their considerable promise.

Beyond Caloric Restriction: Toward Metabolic Precision

As the science of aging advances at a remarkable pace, researchers continue to discover innovative methods that harness the powerful benefits of caloric restriction (CR) and intermittent fasting (IF) without requiring burdensome long-term dietary commitments. Among the most exciting breakthroughs emerging in this dynamic field is the fasting-mimicking diet (FMD), developed by longevity researcher Valter Longo. The FMD is a carefully structured nutritional program designed to replicate the beneficial effects of fasting while providing strategically balanced, limited caloric intake. Typically lasting five days, it gently transitions the body into a fasting-like state, effectively reducing insulin levels, promoting metabolic flexibility, and activating autophagy—the body's natural and beneficial cellular recycling process. Unlike more demanding fasting approaches, FMD achieves metabolic rejuvenation and activation of essential cellular repair mechanisms without the challenges or discomfort often associated with prolonged fasting. For those intimidated or discouraged by continuous fasting regimens, the FMD offers a scientifically validated, practical pathway to sustainably and comfortably experience fasting's benefits.

However, dietary innovations like FMD represent only part of a broader and exciting evolution toward highly personalized, precision-based longevity interventions. Intriguing emerging research highlights considerable variability in responses to CR and IF, shaped significantly by factors such as genetic predispositions, the unique composition of one's microbiome, and individual metabolic histories. Picture two friends embarking on identical fasting protocols: one might experience remarkable improvements in metabolic health, feeling energized and healthier, while the other may notice only modest changes. Such vivid examples underscore why future longevity strategies will likely shift increasingly toward customized interventions. By carefully integrating tailored dietary approaches, meticulous biomarker monitoring, and strategic use of controlled metabolic stressors, researchers and healthcare practitioners are beginning to craft personalized longevity plans designed specifically for each person's distinctive biological makeup.

Moreover, the scientific community's understanding of aging is undergoing a fundamental transformation as it acknowledges how periodic metabolic stress fosters robust cellular resilience. Instead of continuously promoting an environment of caloric abundance, future public health guidance may increasingly embrace strategic nutritional challenges, intended to activate internal repair mechanisms and adaptive longevity pathways. These periodic fasting episodes mirror ancestral cycles of feast and famine, a rhythm that historically sharpened metabolic resilience and efficiency. Ponder how these patterns echo the lives of our ancestors who regularly faced periods of scarcity, emerging healthier and more resilient as a result.

As researchers continue refining these insights, the ultimate challenge will be translating sophisticated scientific discoveries into practical, everyday applications.

Embracing CR and IF through precision-based strategies represents a major shift in nutrition and longevity science, aligning closely with the body's inherent adaptive processes. Rather than obsessively counting calories or pursuing fleeting dietary trends, these targeted interventions activate essential cellular repair systems, enhance metabolic flexibility, and mitigate risks associated with metabolic and age-related diseases. Practical measures—such as slightly reducing daily eating windows, incorporating periodic fasting intervals, or strategically adjusting meal timing—can collectively yield substantial and lasting benefits. Even small yet consistent shifts in dietary habits can yield meaningful improvements, supporting sustained metabolic function and cognitive acuity—both essential for preserving autonomy and lifelong health.

CHAPTER 8

Beyond Rest: Sleep's Secret Role in Longevity and Health

"Sleep is the golden chain that ties health and our bodies together."
—THOMAS DEKKER

Amid the relentless momentum of daily life, where productivity frequently overshadows rest, sleep silently fades into the margins. Society applauds ceaseless activity, perpetual connectivity, and tireless ambition, yet emerging research underscores the essential role of sleep—not only for immediate well-being, but as a cornerstone for enduring vitality and longevity. Sleep is far from passive. Instead, it actively repairs our bodies, rejuvenates our minds, and renews essential physiological functions. Even modestly reducing our sleep can steadily accelerate aging, gradually increasing vulnerability to chronic diseases and diminishing our life expectancy.

Historically, we thought of sleep simply as a way to recover from daily fatigue. Today, groundbreaking science has radically reshaped this view, highlighting sleep as a key determinant of both healthspan and lifespan. Researchers now emphasize that quality sleep is essential for maintaining healthy cells, supporting clear thinking, balancing metabolism, strengthening immunity, and preserving hormonal harmony. Together, these elements powerfully influence how well and how long we live.

Nevertheless, despite the compelling evidence, restful sleep remains one of modern life's most compromised habits. From stressful commutes and extended office hours to scrolling on phones late into the night, contemporary routines quietly chip away at our precious sleep, eroding its quality and duration. Chronic sleep deficiencies have become widespread, incrementally weakening our health.

In the following pages, we'll explore how achieving optimal sleep shapes long-term health, strengthening well-being and enriching overall quality of life. Sleep is perhaps the most underestimated pillar of longevity—often overlooked despite its far-reaching impact on nearly every aspect of our biology. By examining how restorative sleep slows aging, protects cognitive and metabolic functions, and maintains physiological balance, we begin to appreciate sleep not just as a necessity, but as an essential act of self-care. To truly understand sleep's understated yet transformative influence, we must delve deeper into the quiet mysteries that unfold each night, enriching every aspect of our lives.

Understanding Sleep: Foundations of Restoration and Brain Health

Sleep is a familiar yet deeply complex process, vital for preserving health and longevity. Each night, our body and brain cycle through distinct sleep stages, each fulfilling critical restorative roles. Among these stages, deep sleep (slow-wave sleep) and rapid eye movement (REM) sleep are particularly essential, supporting physical renewal, cognitive function, and emotional well-being.

Deep sleep primarily occurs during the first half of the night and is marked by slow, high-amplitude brain waves. In this stage, muscles relax, heart rate and blood pressure decrease, and growth hormone secretion peaks. These physiological changes promote extensive cellular repair and rejuvenation. Additionally, deep sleep plays a crucial role in maintaining immune function, repairing tissues, and optimizing energy metabolism—factors central to longevity. Equally significant is deep sleep's role in activating the brain's glymphatic system, a specialized network that efficiently clears harmful neurotoxic substances like beta-amyloid and tau proteins, safeguarding brain health.

Even small disruptions in deep sleep can significantly impair this cleansing process, increasing the risk of cognitive decline and diseases such as Alzheimer's. Beyond detoxification, deep sleep fosters neuroplasticity by stimulating the release of neurotrophic factors, notably brain-derived neurotrophic factor (BDNF). These factors support neuron survival, neurogenesis, and cognitive resilience. Each night's recalibration consolidates memories, enhances mental clarity, and boosts creativity—critical for sustaining long-term cognitive health.

In contrast, REM sleep predominates in the latter half of the night, underpinning essential cognitive processes such as memory consolidation, learning, and emotional regulation. During REM sleep, the brain actively reorganizes neural pathways, strengthening important memories and eliminating irrelevant information. This mental housekeeping is vital for emotional balance and cognitive strength, both essential for enduring health and vitality.

The delicate balance between deep and REM sleep cycles is governed by our internal biological clock, known as the circadian rhythm. Influenced primarily by the cycles of natural daylight and darkness, the circadian rhythm synchronizes sleep-wake patterns, body temperature, hormone production, and metabolism. Disruptions to this rhythm—commonly experienced with shift work, frequent travel, or irregular sleep patterns—can accelerate aging, impair immunity, and heighten vulnerability to chronic illness.

Another core component of sleep science is sleep homeostasis, the body's balance between wakefulness and the increasing pressure to sleep. This balance is mediated by biochemical signals like adenosine, a neuromodulator accumulating in the brain during wakefulness. Rising adenosine levels trigger sleepiness, intensifying the natural drive for rest and facilitating a smooth transition into sleep. Disrupting this balance through inadequate or irregular sleep leads to fatigue, cognitive impairment, hormonal disturbances, and accelerated aging.

By understanding these foundational mechanisms—deep sleep, REM sleep, circadian rhythms, and sleep homeostasis—we gain deeper insight into how quality sleep shapes physical health, cognitive function, emotional well-being, and longevity. Prioritizing sleep ensures vital processes such as glymphatic clearance and neuroplasticity continue effectively, slowing cognitive decline, bolstering resilience, and promoting a longer, healthier life.

Hormonal and Circadian Regulation by Sleep

Sleep effectively regulates hormonal balance, a crucial aspect of metabolic function. Hormones perform a meticulously choreographed dance, requiring precise synchronization to maintain bodily harmony. Disrupted sleep—whether due to insufficient duration or diminished quality—can disturb this hormonal rhythm, causing elevations in stress hormones like cortisol, impairments in insulin sensitivity, and instability in appetite-regulating hormones such as leptin and ghrelin. Leptin, predominantly produced by fat cells, signals satiety to the brain when energy stores are sufficient. Ghrelin, originating mainly in the stomach, stimulates appetite when the body requires energy. Disruptions in this delicate balance result in impaired eating behaviors, weight gain, and heightened susceptibility to obesity, diabetes, and cardiovascular disease.

Beyond hormonal harmony, sleep aligns physiological processes with innate circadian rhythms. Frequent disruptions to these natural rhythms—due to repeated travel across time zones, late-night screen exposure, or irregular shift work—can induce chronic inflammation and accelerate biological aging. In contrast, tailoring daily routines to align with one's personal chronotype, be it "early bird" or "night owl," enhances physiological resilience and supports long-term health and longevity.

Additionally, sleep enhances immune system function, sharpening immunological defenses and reinforcing immune memory. Recent research underscores the significance of quality sleep in enhancing vaccine effectiveness and resilience against infections. Even outward appearance benefits significantly from recuperative sleep, as nighttime surges in growth hormone stimulate tissue repair, skin regeneration, and collagen synthesis—rejuvenating appearance and accelerating wound healing. Furthermore, the reciprocal relationship between sleep quality and the microbiome highlights deeper interconnections between rest and metabolic wellness.

Innovative developments in genetics and wearable sleep-monitoring technologies now enable unparalleled personalization in optimizing sleep. Advanced wearable trackers and AI-driven sleep applications offer detailed insights into individual sleep patterns. Personalized genetic analyses further empower tailored strategies for deeper and more restorative sleep. Making restful sleep a priority and aligning lifestyle habits accordingly constitutes an essential, proactive investment in lifelong well-being, enhancing not only nightly revitalization but enriching every waking moment.

The Foundations—Sleep and the Biology of Aging

Sleep exerts a far-reaching influence on aging, orchestrating nightly restorative processes that renew and repair cells at the deepest biological levels. Essential mechanisms shaping biological age and resilience—telomere maintenance, DNA repair, epigenetic regulation, and mitochondrial preservation—depend intimately on restful sleep.

Telomeres act as internal clocks, marking cellular age by gradually shortening with each cell division until triggering cellular senescence and visible signs of aging. Consistent, high-quality sleep substantially slows this telomere shortening by reducing systemic inflammation and oxidative stress, factors known to accelerate telomere erosion. Conversely, chronic sleep deprivation speeds telomere loss by heightening inflammatory responses and oxidative damage, underscoring the crucial protective role regular restorative sleep plays in aging.

Sleep plays a crucial role in cellular health by meticulously safeguarding DNA integrity against daily damage from metabolic processes, environmental toxins, and ultraviolet radiation. Specialized repair mechanisms—particularly base excision repair (BER) and nucleotide excision repair (NER)—peak during deep, restorative sleep, significantly enhancing the activity of vital DNA repair enzymes like poly(ADP-ribose) polymerase-1 (PARP-1). Without this nightly maintenance, genetic damage accumulates swiftly, accelerating aging and increasing susceptibility to chronic diseases.

Epigenetic regulation—chemical modifications influencing gene expression without altering genetic sequences—is markedly shaped by sleep quality. Chronic sleep loss accelerates epigenetic aging through detrimental DNA methylation patterns, especially hypermethylation of genes associated with metabolism, stress responses, and inflammation. In contrast, regular, restorative sleep preserves youthful epigenetic patterns via beneficial histone modifications and finely-tuned microRNA expression, reinforcing optimal cellular function and longevity.

Additionally, groundbreaking research links sleep directly to mitochondrial health—the cellular energy powerhouses whose efficiency naturally declines with age. Sleep revitalizes mitochondria by stimulating mitochondrial biogenesis—the creation of new mitochondria—and enhancing mitochondrial repair through transcription factors such as PGC-1α, a protein that regulates energy production and mitochondrial function. Maintaining mitochondrial integrity through consistent sleep ensures continuous cellular energy production essential for overall vitality and sustained longevity.

Sleep and Metabolic Health—Supporting Hormonal and Cardiovascular Well-being

Sleep actively supports metabolic balance and cardiovascular wellness through nuanced hormonal adjustments. Disruptions to sleep patterns elevate chronic metabolic and cardiovascular risks by destabilizing appetite-regulating hormones, impairing insulin sensitivity, increasing cortisol production, and intensifying systemic inflammation. Dietary choices significantly impact sleep quality and metabolic outcomes. Diets rich in lean proteins and dietary fiber enhance restful sleep by stabilizing blood glucose and promoting a balanced gut microbiome. Aligning meal timing with circadian rhythms improves insulin sensitivity, cholesterol profiles, triglyceride levels, and reduces inflammation, thereby strengthening cardiovascular function. Ultimately, harmonizing consistent sleep practices, genetic insights, and supportive dietary habits deeply enhances metabolic and cardiovascular health, affirming sleep as a cornerstone of lifelong wellness and longevity.

The Microbiome and Sleep—A Reciprocal Relationship

Within each of us resides a vibrant and diverse community of microorganisms known as the microbiome, with a particularly rich presence in the gut. This microbial ecosystem plays a significant role in shaping our health, mood, and quality of sleep. Through the gut-brain axis, these microbes communicate actively with the brain, influencing emotional well-being, metabolism, immunity, and sleep-wake cycles.

Beneficial gut bacteria, such as *Lactobacillus* and *Bifidobacterium*, facilitate the conversion of dietary tryptophan into serotonin, a neurotransmitter that promotes deep, restorative sleep. Additionally, the microbiome contributes to the production of gamma-aminobutyric acid (GABA), a compound that calms brain activity, alleviates anxiety, and enhances sleep quality.

However, when the microbiome is out of balance—known as dysbiosis—it contributes to harmful bacterial overgrowth. This leads to an increase in inflammatory markers like cytokines IL-6 and TNF-alpha, which heighten stress responses and impair sleep. Dysbiosis is a key player in the development of chronic conditions, including cardiovascular disease, diabetes, and cognitive decline. The cycle of poor sleep and a disrupted microbiome only perpetuates systemic inflammation and metabolic dysfunction.

By understanding this reciprocal relationship between the microbiome and sleep, we can adopt holistic strategies to enhance health and support longevity.

Enhancing Sleep Through Lifestyle—Nutrition, Movement, and Practical Strategies

Lifestyle choices—especially those related to nutrition and physical activity—have a major impact on sleep quality, particularly as we age. Thoughtful adjustments in these areas can help sustain deep, restorative sleep, which is essential for long-term well-being.

Nutrition plays a pivotal role in sleep. Consuming lean proteins like poultry, fish, eggs, and legumes provides sleep-promoting amino acids, including tryptophan (which converts into serotonin) and glycine (which helps reduce core body temperature). High-fiber foods such as oats, fruits, vegetables, nuts, and whole grains stabilize blood sugar levels overnight, reducing sleep disturbances. In contrast, high-fat, processed, or fried foods consumed late in the day can impair sleep quality. Healthy fats, such as those found in olive oil, avocados, and nuts, consumed earlier in the day, help maintain stable blood sugar and provide sustained energy through the night, supporting better sleep.

Physical activity plays a vital role in promoting restorative sleep. Resistance training, for example, stimulates the release of growth hormone, vital for tissue repair during sleep, while aerobic activities help to regulate circadian rhythms and deepen rest.

Creating the right environment for sleep can further enhance its quality. Maintaining a cool bedroom (60-67°F) optimizes melatonin production, aiding in sleep initiation. Limiting evening exposure to artificial blue light from electronic devices helps maintain natural melatonin rhythms. Establishing a consistent sleep routine that incorporates relaxation techniques—such as gentle stretching, mindfulness meditation, or deep-breathing exercises—can effectively lower stress, ease sleep onset, and improve overall sleep quality.

By intentionally combining dietary adjustments, physical activity, and thoughtful bedtime strategies, we can create the optimal conditions for rejuvenating sleep, which will have far-reaching benefits for mood, resilience, and vitality.

The Quiet Architect of Life: Sleep's Role in Shaping Our Future

Sleep is far more than a passive nightly occurrence—it's a deliberate investment in our long-term health, cognitive clarity, and emotional resilience. Each night, deep restorative sleep resets our bodies and minds, replenishing energy, strengthening resilience, and renewing our capacity to face each new day with clarity. Sleep touches every aspect of our biology—strengthening cellular integrity, bolstering immune function, and sharpening brain performance. Prioritizing recuperative sleep is like equipping ourselves with emotional armor, enabling us to calmly navigate life's daily stresses and challenges.

By adopting practical strategies and personalized approaches explored earlier, we can actively harness sleep as a powerful tool for lifelong health. Advances in sleep-monitoring technologies now offer individualized optimization, tailored to our unique genetic profiles and real-time physiological responses, making restful sleep increasingly achievable for everyone.

In the final analysis, prioritizing sleep enhances physical repair, mental resilience, cognitive function, and our overall quality of life. As scientific consensus continues to grow, sleep emerges as an empowering, foundational pillar for sustained health—a revitalizing nightly ritual that enriches daily experience and fortifies long-term well-being.

CHAPTER 9

Mental Resilience and Stress Management: Cultivating Inner Strength for Longevity

"The greatest weapon against stress is our ability to choose one thought over another."
—WILLIAM JAMES

In the quest for longevity, the mind often remains in the shadows, rarely receiving the spotlight it genuinely deserves. Psychological attributes such as mental resilience, emotional stability, and skillful stress management form indispensable pillars of enduring wellness—often subtle but always powerful. These internal strengths shape our health, influencing both the quality of our lives and their duration.

Mental resilience—the capacity to adapt fluidly to adversity and swiftly regain equilibrium—functions like a flexible shield, bending without breaking under life's relentless pressures. Rather than fracturing during turbulent times, the resilient mind navigates challenges with poise, preserving emotional harmony and safeguarding physical health. Complementing this resilience, emotional stability nurtures optimism, cultivates gratitude, and fortifies meaningful social bonds, protecting us from premature aging and chronic illness.

Encouragingly, psychological strength isn't exclusive to a fortunate few naturally predisposed to resilience; instead, it can flourish within anyone through consistent, approachable practices. Simple, evidence-based habits such as relaxation exercises, gratitude journaling, fostering deep relationships, and cognitive reframing gradually reinforce emotional fortitude while steadily diminishing stress. Integrating these routines into daily life not only enriches our everyday experiences but also adds meaningful years to our lifespan.

The Scientific Foundations of Mental Resilience, Stress Management, and Longevity

On biological and neurological levels, persistent stress accelerates aging and disease progression. While brief episodes of stress can sharpen focus and temporarily boost performance, prolonged stress significantly undermines physical and cognitive health, primarily due to chronically elevated cortisol levels. Sustained cortisol secretion is associated with accelerated telomere shortening—the progressive erosion of protective chromosome caps—which ultimately leads cells into a state of senescence. Senescent cells, in turn, secrete pro-inflammatory factors, fostering chronic inflammation and heightening susceptibility to cardiovascular disease, diabetes, and certain cancers.

Additionally, chronic stress impairs mitochondrial function, diminishing the cell's ability to produce energy effectively. This dysfunction increases oxidative stress and disrupts metabolic homeostasis, potentially leading to metabolic disorders and accelerating the aging process. Persistent cortisol elevation further dysregulates the hypothalamic-pituitary-adrenal (HPA) axis—the body's primary stress-response system—resulting in immune suppression and sustained inflammation. These cumulative physiological disruptions constitute what is known as "allostatic load," the long-term biological burden of chronic stress.

From a neurological standpoint, continuous stress exposure damages crucial brain regions essential for cognitive clarity and emotional regulation. Chronic stress notably reduces hippocampal volume, impairing memory and cognitive abilities and elevating vulnerability to neurodegenerative diseases such as Alzheimer's. Moreover, extended stress exposure decreases levels of brain-derived neurotrophic factor (BDNF), a vital protein supporting neuronal survival, synaptic plasticity, and cognitive adaptability.

Fortunately, resilience-promoting practices actively leverage neuroplasticity, enabling the brain to reorganize and strengthen neural connections essential for emotional regulation and cognitive flexibility. Functional MRI studies illustrate that structured cognitive-behavioral interventions and consistent mindfulness practices significantly decrease hyperactivity in the amygdala—the brain's primary stress-response center—while simultaneously strengthening the prefrontal cortex, a region crucial for emotional control and decision-making. Thus, actively cultivating psychological resilience mitigates stress-induced physiological damage, contributing to enhanced longevity and improved overall health.

Resilience as a Protective Factor

Resilience acts as a protective buffer—not by eliminating stressors but by equipping people to effectively navigate life's inevitable adversities. Conceptually, resilience resembles a muscle, strengthened specifically through encountering and overcoming challenges. Those with greater resilience handle life's stresses more adeptly, recovering emotional equilibrium swiftly and maintaining consistently lower cortisol levels. Such adaptability bolsters immune function, reduces systemic inflammation, and protects cardiovascular and cognitive health.

Neurologically, resilience directly counters chronic stress's damaging effects. By preserving and enhancing levels of crucial brain proteins such as BDNF, resilience fosters robust neuroplasticity. This neuroprotective capacity supports neuron survival and growth, indirectly facilitating neurogenesis and cognitive flexibility, thereby reducing the risk of cognitive impairment and dementia. Furthermore, resilience's modulation of inflammatory responses contributes substantially to maintaining overall brain integrity and cognitive function, underscoring its critical role in longevity and quality of life.

The Role of Mind-Body Practices

Mind-body methods—including meditation, present-moment awareness, and gratitude—actively engage the brain's extraordinary capacity for neuroplasticity, the innate ability to reorganize and adapt based on experience. By directing attention to the present moment and non-judgmentally observing thoughts, sensations, and emotions, these practices reshape neural connections. Over time, this deliberate and mindful engagement reduces cortisol levels and fortifies neural pathways crucial to emotional balance. Robust research consistently highlights measurable health benefits from these techniques, such as enhanced heart rate variability—a key marker of stress resilience—and improved mitochondrial efficiency, vital for cellular energy and sustained health.

Integrating these mindful strategies into daily routines gradually transforms negative thought patterns into more constructive perspectives, diminishing psychological tension and physiological stress responses. While individually beneficial, these practices gain additional strength during periods of heightened stress or emotional turmoil when combined with professional, evidence-based approaches such as cognitive-behavioral therapy (CBT). CBT provides structured tools to manage emotional and cognitive challenges, complementing self-guided meditation practices. Embracing professional guidance alongside personal efforts underscores a proactive commitment to sustained mental, emotional, and physical well-being.

Physical Activity, Relaxation, and Breathing Techniques

Physical activity represents a powerful, natural antidote to stress, linking bodily movement with emotional equilibrium. Even simple activities—like morning walks, leisurely cycling, or gentle yoga stretches—stimulate the release of endorphins, your body's intrinsic mood enhancers. Regular exercise not only alleviates anxiety but also bolsters cardiovascular health, enhances immune function, and encourages neurogenesis—the formation of new neurons. Over time, these consistent physical practices build lasting stamina and increase psychological flexibility.

Complementing movement, relaxation techniques offer accessible yet effective tools for managing daily pressures. Practices such as deep breathing exercises, progressive muscle relaxation, and guided visualization activate the parasympathetic nervous system, the body's inherent calming mechanism. These approachable methods serve as personal sanctuaries, always available to restore emotional balance amidst life's inevitable challenges.

Further supporting resilience, thoughtful boundary-setting safeguards mental resources. Imagine boundaries as protective fences around your psychological reserves, empowering you to handle demands thoughtfully and preventing feelings of overwhelm. Prioritizing intentional self-care through clear boundaries preserves mental clarity, emotional reserves, and adaptive capacity.

Cumulative Benefits for Longevity

When integrated, scientifically validated practices—including mindfulness, gratitude, regular exercise, intentional boundary-setting, structured relaxation techniques, and professional support—offer cumulative benefits. Collectively, these behaviors positively influence biological aging by protecting telomere integrity, optimizing mitochondrial function, and reducing inflammation. Cognitively, they cultivate inner balance and mental agility, equipping us to face life's inevitable challenges with clarity, confidence, and optimism.

Together, these habitual practices form a cohesive strategy for sustained longevity. Beyond alleviating immediate stress, they actively nurture biological adaptability, safeguard against age-related illnesses, and support enduring mental and physical strength.

The Mind as a Guardian of Health and Longevity

Mental resilience and skillful stress management constitute foundational pillars of lifelong wellness. The intricate interplay between mind and body ensures that psychological well-being positively influences physical health and overall lifespan. Cultivating adaptability and proactively addressing stressors builds a robust internal defense against chronic disease, cognitive decline, and premature aging.

While unmanaged stress accelerates cellular aging, heightens inflammation, and hastens cognitive deterioration, resilience reframes adversity into meaningful opportunities for growth and insight. Mental flexibility, enriching relationships, consistent physical activity, and mindful awareness collectively form a robust, protective framework safeguarding long-term health.

Prioritizing emotional balance and mental strength enriches life outside the bounds of longevity alone. A clarity of purpose, authentic connections, and personal fulfillment naturally arise from these intentional, holistic practices, enhancing every life experience. Longevity thus evolves beyond the accumulation of years into a conscious commitment to meaningful engagement, genuine relationships, and sustained emotional—and consequently physical—resilience.

CHAPTER 10

Emotional and Spiritual Wellness: A Holistic Approach to Aging

"It is only with the heart that one can see rightly; what is essential is invisible to the eye."
—ANTOINE DE SAINT-EXUPÉRY, THE LITTLE PRINCE

A truly fulfilling life, enriched in both length and depth, calls for more than attention to physical health. While discussions of longevity typically center around nutrition, exercise, and sleep, underpinning these visible elements are psychological and spiritual dimensions, deeply shaping our happiness, resilience, and overall sense of meaning. These often-overlooked foundations do more than enhance daily experiences; they protect us against chronic diseases and equip us to navigate life's inevitable peaks and valleys with grace.

Psychological stability, purposeful living, and meaningful relationships collectively elevate not only the quality of our lives but their duration as well. In this chapter, we journey into the scientific landscape underpinning emotional and spiritual wellness, uncover measurable impacts on physical health, and provide practical strategies to incorporate these vital dimensions into the rhythm of your everyday experience—crafting a comprehensive, personalized blueprint for longevity.

The Science of Emotional and Spiritual Health

Emotional and spiritual wellness extend beyond abstract concepts—they have tangible impacts on biological systems vital for healthy aging. The field of psychoneuroimmunology, which investigates the interplay among emotional states, nervous system function, and immune response, demonstrates how our internal emotional climate can shape physical well-being. Positive emotional states—such as gratitude, compassion, and optimism—are associated with improved metabolic regulation, including better control of blood glucose levels. Research demonstrates that positive affect is associated with lower cortisol levels, enhanced immune responses, and superior cardiovascular functioning. Positive emotional states also correlate with increased heart rate variability (HRV), a measure of autonomic balance linked to reduced mortality and lower chronic disease risk.

Neuropeptides, especially oxytocin, released during meaningful social interactions, play an essential role in regulating stress responses, enhancing social bonds, and building resilience. Oxytocin has been shown to reduce inflammation, buffer stress responses, and moderate hypothalamic-pituitary-adrenal (HPA) axis activity, thereby supporting effective coping mechanisms during extended periods of stress.

Neuroscientific research employing electroencephalograms (EEGs) and functional magnetic resonance imaging (fMRI) further reveals the neural benefits of spiritual practices. Mindfulness meditation and contemplative prayer reliably shift brain-wave patterns toward states of calm attentiveness, engaging and strengthening key areas like the anterior cingulate cortex and prefrontal cortex—regions central to emotional regulation and cognitive control. Long-term meditation practice has even been associated with increased cortical thickness, particularly within brain regions linked to emotional processing and cognitive functioning.

Longitudinal epidemiological research reinforces the health advantages of sustained spiritual involvement. Significant observational studies connect regular spiritual or religious participation with reduced mortality rates in older adults. Additional studies consistently associate spiritual practices with decreased inflammatory biomarkers, such as C-reactive protein (CRP) and interleukin-6 (IL-6). Mindfulness-based stress reduction techniques have been shown to effectively increase telomerase activity, crucial for maintaining telomere length and mitigating cellular aging.

Epigenetic studies exploring how lifestyle and emotional states influence gene expression provide additional compelling evidence. Emerging research indicates mindfulness and similar practices trigger beneficial gene expression changes, notably reducing nuclear factor kappa B (NF-kB) signaling—a prominent inflammatory pathway involved in aging and chronic disease.

Creative activities bridge emotional and spiritual domains uniquely, offering complementary health benefits. Artistic endeavors such as painting, writing, and music-making stimulate dopaminergic reward pathways in the brain, enhance psychological flexibility, and facilitate emotional expression. Neuroimaging research shows that creative expression strengthens connectivity within the default mode network, a neural network integral to self-reflection, emotional regulation, and cognitive adaptability. These forms of creative engagement effectively buffer against stress, significantly contributing to emotional stability and cognitive resilience.

Taken together, this scientific evidence highlights emotional and spiritual health as key determinants of biological resilience and healthy aging. Their influences reach beyond subjective experiences, directly impacting physiological processes and significantly enhancing the quality, grace, and capacity of aging.

The Lifelong Journey Toward Inner Harmony

Psychological and spiritual health dynamically evolve throughout every stage of life, adapting to shifting challenges and opportunities. During childhood and adolescence, cultivating emotional intelligence, self-awareness, and open communication provides a strong foundation for lifelong adaptability. Imagine these early psychological skills as a carefully constructed scaffold, built through supportive relationships, empowering young people to confidently navigate life's uncertainties.

Adulthood brings increasing responsibilities such as careers, family commitments, and caregiving roles. These responsibilities present formidable challenges but also meaningful opportunities for personal growth. Such pivotal moments often inspire deeper reflection, clarify core values, and reconnect us with renewed purpose. Actively integrating resilience practices like regular meditation or mindful creativity during these demanding years fosters balance, optimism, and mental clarity amid life's complexities.

In later years, the quest for deeper meaning typically intensifies, prompting contemplation of legacy, purpose, and the significance of social connections. Practices such as gratitude journaling, introspection, acceptance, and spiritual reflection—including nurturing a personal relationship with God—serve as powerful anchors for internal stability. Continued social engagement and lifelong learning preserve a sense of purpose, counteracting loneliness and challenges associated with decreased independence. Supportive relationships, spiritual nourishment, and an enduringly curious mindset ensure that later life remains psychologically vibrant, meaningful, and rewarding.

Across each life stage, emotional and spiritual wellness support inner stability, enrich personal connections, and continually deepen our appreciation of life's unfolding journey.

Paths to Fulfillment in the Face of Adversity

Life inevitably presents challenges that test our psychological and spiritual resilience. Acknowledging and effectively addressing these obstacles is crucial for sustained well-being. Chronic anxiety and unresolved emotional trauma, for example, can undermine both mental equilibrium and physical health. Like an untreated wound that festers, persistent psychological distress erodes immune function and accelerates aging. Seeking professional support through therapy, counseling, or intentional reflective practices nurtures emotional healing and fosters inner adaptability.

Social isolation, increasingly prevalent today, significantly increases health risks such as depression, cardiovascular disease, and cognitive decline. Deliberately cultivating meaningful relationships with family, friends, or community groups rekindles warmth and a comforting sense of belonging, significantly alleviating loneliness and bolstering emotional and physical resilience.

Consistent participation in religious services and communal worship provides meaningful psychological comfort that extends beyond companionship. Shared rituals, prayers, songs, and collective silence strengthen interpersonal bonds, fortify emotional resilience, and foster a sense of collective identity. For those whose beliefs might limit participation in traditional spiritual practices, spirituality transcends conventional boundaries, offering diverse pathways to fulfillment. Immersion in nature, creative activities, or acts of kindness and service provide potent avenues for spiritual enrichment, aligning authentically with individual values and beliefs.

Practical Strategies for Cultivating Emotional and Spiritual Wellness in Longevity Practices

Emotional and spiritual wellness constitute foundational pillars of a purposeful, enduring life. Incorporating these dimensions into everyday routines involves intentionally selecting activities that enhance psychological adaptability, deepen spiritual connections, and clarify life's purpose. Mindfulness and meditation offer accessible avenues to emotional balance and mental clarity. Even dedicating just a few quiet moments daily to meditation significantly reduces stress, eases anxiety, uplifts mood, and sharpens cognitive faculties. Embedding mindfulness into routine experiences—such as conscious breathing or savoring nature's beauty—transforms ordinary moments into tranquil, restorative interludes.

Practicing gratitude further reinforces psychological stability. Keeping a daily gratitude journal, reflecting briefly on positive experiences, or performing small acts of kindness can shift one's outlook, deepening emotional resilience and personal satisfaction. Building robust social connections through regular community activities like shared meals, group exercise, meditation gatherings, or volunteering fosters meaningful bonds, reduces isolation, and enhances psychological flexibility.

Consistent engagement in worship can significantly enhance spiritual well-being. Inspiring sermons encourage thoughtful reflection, prayers offer comfort and clarity, and spiritually meaningful music touches the heart, creating moments of inner peace and renewal. For those who embrace faith, regular worship provides genuine opportunities to experience a personal connection with the divine, fostering spiritual growth and emotional strength. Cultivating a relationship with God adds depth and meaning to these experiences, offering guidance, comfort, and a deep sense of purpose. Over time, this dedicated commitment fosters spiritual maturity and nurtures a harmonious inner life.

Integrating these practical approaches into daily living anchors emotional and spiritual wellness within longevity practices, shifting the focus from merely extending lifespan to enriching it with intention, depth, and fulfillment.

CHAPTER 11

The Pleasure Principle: Sexual Intimacy

I love you without knowing how, or when, or from where. I love you straightforwardly, without complexities or pride."
—Pablo Neruda

Sex itself remains widely misunderstood, often dismissed as mere indulgence or trivialized as fleeting gratification. This common misperception overlooks its essential role and the meaningful combination of emotional closeness and physical connection, and how they influence longevity. Beyond momentary satisfaction, sexual intimacy steadies us, reducing stress, relieving loneliness, and deepening our connections during life's inevitable challenges. Over time, these beneficial effects accumulate, reinforcing relationships, and resilience necessary for lasting fulfillment.

Sex is more than pleasure—it holds profound power. Consider sexual intimacy as nature's prescription for well-being, quietly nurturing emotional bonds and strengthening health.

In this chapter, we move beyond familiar assumptions, exploring how passion, closeness, hormonal balance, and overall health intertwine in surprising ways. Pleasure provides a natural and meaningful pathway toward sustained health and longevity. By intentionally cultivating sexual intimacy, we invest in our longevity.

Fire and Foundation: Understanding Sex and Intimacy

Sex and intimacy, though closely linked, serve distinctly complementary roles.

Sex is dynamic. It vividly expresses physical desire, connects deeply with emotional affection, and provides immediate yet enduring benefits. Beyond pleasure alone, sexual activity significantly enhances overall well-being, lowering stress, decreasing cortisol, and reinforcing hormonal balance. These positive effects swiftly improve mood, ease anxiety, and rejuvenate both body and mind.

Intimacy offers the steady, supportive counterpart, developing gradually from trust, vulnerability, and genuine emotional closeness. Often subtle yet deeply meaningful, intimacy emerges through comforting embraces, after challenging days, quiet conversations filled with understanding, or shared laughter over life's unexpected moments. These interactions anchor relationships, providing stability amid life's uncertainties.

When sex and intimacy harmonize, these two elements have the ability to strengthen human connection and activate biochemical responses that reinforce closeness and health. Their synergy is essential, creating companionships rich with happiness, resilience, and satisfaction. Recognizing and nurturing the interplay between sex and intimacy deepens emotional bonding and sustains lasting passion.

The Science of Sexual Health: The Hidden Link Between Sexual Intimacy and Longevity

Sexual health significantly influences overall wellness, enhancing physical vitality, emotional balance, and longevity. Like regular exercise and balanced nutrition, an active and fulfilling sex life offers substantial health benefits supported by extensive research.

At a cellular level, sexual activity preserves essential biological structures—particularly telomeres, the protective caps at chromosome ends. Telomeres shorten naturally with aging, a process accelerated by chronic stress and inflammation, increasing susceptibility to cardiovascular disease, cancer, and dementia. Recent studies, such as those published in Psychoneuroendocrinology, suggest that regular sexual activity significantly slows telomere attrition, maintaining genomic integrity.

Additionally, emerging research, such as the recent CAPLIFE study, reveals a compelling link between ejaculation frequency and prostate cancer risk. Men who ejaculate frequently show a notably lower risk of prostate cancer, especially in aggressive or advanced forms. Regular ejaculation thus appears to offer a simple, natural approach to potentially reducing prostate cancer risk, underscoring sex's role in preventive health care.

Sex stimulates beneficial hormonal responses, temporarily boosting growth hormone production, which in turn promotes cellular regeneration, muscle maintenance, metabolic efficiency, and skin elasticity. It elevates testosterone and estrogen levels, vital for maintaining bone density, cardiovascular health, and libido.

Cognitively, sexual activity increases cerebral circulation, delivering nutrients and oxygen to brain regions essential for memory, clarity, and mental agility. Prolactin, released post-orgasm, improves sleep quality, crucial for cognitive restoration and protection against neurodegenerative conditions such as Alzheimer's.

Sex alone can temporarily boost immune function by increasing immunoglobulin A (IgA), an antibody essential for mucosal barrier defense, potentially reducing susceptibility to infections. Additionally, sex's analgesic effects, driven by endorphin release, offer relief from chronic pain conditions like migraines, arthritis, and menstrual discomfort. Sexual activity naturally stabilizes mood by releasing neurotransmitters such as dopamine and serotonin. Dopamine elevates pleasure and motivation, while serotonin gently soothes anxiety, fostering emotional balance like rays of sunshine dispersing clouds. Oxytocin, often called the "bonding hormone," is notably elevated during sexual experiences, quietly reinforcing human connection. Such enriched bonds act as a buffer against social isolation, providing personal stability, and relational resilience.

When emotional intimacy accompanies sex, it unlocks distinct, additional health benefits. Sex with intimacy further intensifies the release of hormones like oxytocin and vasopressin, fostering deeper bonding, trust, and relationship satisfaction. These enriched interactions reduce stress and its negative health impacts. Moreover, sexual intimacy triggers more pronounced elevations of neurotransmitters such as dopamine and serotonin, enhancing mood and resilience against anxiety, depression, and cognitive decline. It also strongly reinforces interpersonal bonds, reducing loneliness and providing sustained emotional nourishment crucial to psychological health.

While sex offers immediate physiological benefits, sexual intimacy provides deeper enduring health advantages and enriches human connection. Prioritizing sexual intimacy represents a scientifically validated approach to lifelong health and well-being.

Sexual Intimacy and Sleep: A Vital Connection

An intriguing yet often-overlooked connection between sexual intimacy and improved sleep has emerged from recent research, highlighting a natural pathway toward better health and greater longevity. Think of sexual intimacy as nature's soothing lullaby, preparing body and mind for restful sleep. Studies confirm that partnered sexual activity significantly improves sleep quality compared to solo experiences, likely due to distinct emotional and hormonal factors.

This enhanced effect appears linked to shared closeness and trust experienced during partnered sexual intimacy, creating an atmosphere conducive to deep relaxation. The presence of a sympathetic partner fosters a sense of safety, amplifying sleep's restorative powers. Quality sleep strengthens immune function, reduces chronic inflammation, and lowers risks associated with cardiovascular diseases and cognitive decline—all vital components of sustained longevity. Sexual intimacy and sleep support each other in a harmonious cycle: intimacy enhances restful sleep, restorative sleep improves health, and improved health, in turn, nurtures sexual intimacy.

Sexual Intimacy and Aging: Life Changes

"Pleasure is the flower that passes; remembrance, the lasting perfume."
—Jean de Boufflers

From youth onward, cultivating a healthy attitude towards sexuality lays a critical foundation for lifelong wellness. Early sexual education acts like planting seeds in the garden of future health, guiding a comfortable embracement of sex and intimacy throughout life.

During midlife, shifts in hormones often redefine sexual intimacy. Men typically experience decreases in testosterone, and women commonly encounter reduced estrogen levels during menopause. These natural hormonal shifts influence sexual intimacy. Rather than indicating decline, these transitions have the potential to invite couples toward greater openness, adaptability, and compassionate communication. These changes can be embraced as opportunities to explore new forms of interpersonal attachment. Sustaining sexual intimacy into later life offers substantial health benefits, including enhanced cardiovascular function, improved cognitive clarity, emotional stability, and reduced risk of depression. Regular affectionate interactions significantly enhance well-being among older adults. By openly addressing aging-related changes in sexual intimacy, couples actively challenge societal stigmas, affirming sex as a flexible and essential component of lifelong emotional and physical health.

Sexual intimacy is a vital evolving element of relationships across the lifespan. While sexual activity provides direct physical health benefits, emotional intimacy nurtures deeper psychological connections, strengthens relationships, and enhances overall quality of life. Prioritizing both enriches lives, fosters enduring bonds, and significantly contributes to longevity and health.

Self-Intimacy: Unlocking Longevity and Wellness Through Physical Pleasure

"The relationship with oneself sets the tone for every other relationship."
—Jane Travis

Intimacy extends beyond connections with others—it originates within oneself. Independent living offers a unique opportunity to deepen physical self-awareness. Thoughtful engagement in physical self-intimacy can unlock substantial emotional, psychological, and physiological rewards, enhancing overall health, longevity, and personal fulfillment.

Physical self-pleasure, though occasionally misunderstood, actually nourishes the body and mind. Consider it mindful self-care—a powerful method to dissolve stress, balance hormones, and elevate one's mood. Scientific research highlights its ability to stimulate beneficial hormonal responses such as dopamine, serotonin, and oxytocin, stabilizing emotions, alleviating anxiety, and sharpening cognitive clarity. Regular physical self-pleasure also improves sleep quality by releasing prolactin, essential for restorative sleep.

Beyond immediate physical sensations, purposeful self-intimacy promotes deeper bodily awareness and acceptance. Incorporating mindfulness practices—such as synchronized breathing exercises, reflective solitude, or guided meditation, enhances these benefits significantly. Intentional self-exploration helps map the landscape of both body and mind, pointing towards future human connections, reducing isolation and improving psychological balance.

Recognizing that physical self-intimacy may not be suitable or comfortable for everyone emphasizes the importance of embracing non-physical intimacy as a valuable alternative. Non-physical self-intimacy flourishes through supportive self-dialogue, thoughtful reflection, and meaningful contemplation, each of which offers comfort and reassurance. Cultivating one's emotional and psychological self enhances authenticity and empathy to others. This encourages friendships, enriches family relationships and engagement with community.

These varied forms of intimacy effectively alleviate loneliness and provide essential warmth and support throughout life's diverse experiences. Self-intimacy involves more than simply replacing partnered connections; it helps reshape how we experience closeness with others, deepening emotional insight and authenticity. By embracing self-intimacy—in physical interactions or reflective solitude—people build resilience, increase self-understanding, and find fulfillment in ways that may surprise them. Ultimately, these intimate experiences enrich life, continuously offering new perspectives and opportunities for personal growth.

The Case for Intentional Sex: Could Prioritizing Sexual Intimacy be Among Life's Most Meaningful Investments?

> *"And the day came when the risk to remain tight in a bud was more painful than the risk it took to blossom."*
> —ANAÏS NIN

Sexual intimacy offers significant benefits beyond immediate pleasure, playing a crucial role in physical health, emotional stability, and overall longevity. Regular sexual intimacy supports immune function, strengthens cardiovascular health, elevates mood, alleviates chronic pain, and promotes restful sleep. Yet despite these substantial advantages, it often slips down the priority list, overshadowed by stress, fatigue, and modern life's constant demands. Many people feel distant, longing for closeness but uncertain how to obtain pleasure amidst relationship difficulties and daily challenges.

What if we regarded sexual intimacy as a nurturing form of self-care, enhancing life quality and deepening interpersonal connections? Intentionally engaging in these activities supports immunity, boosts heart health, and reduces chronic pain, all while fostering restful sleep. Far from an indulgence, sexual intimacy represents a meaningful investment in long-term well-being.

Modern life's busy schedules, digital distractions, and shifting desires frequently sideline sexual intimacy, resulting in loneliness. Without intentional effort, sex can become limited to rare moments when conditions seem ideal. Research consistently demonstrates that couples who consciously nurture their physical connection experience greater emotional strength, deeper relational satisfaction, and reduced relationship stress, even during busy or challenging periods. Deliberate sexual activity doesn't require rigid schedules. Getting to this destination involves self-reflection and conscious actions.

Couples who purposefully maintain closeness often find themselves healthier, physically more resilient, and cognitively sharper. Intentional sexual intimacy transforms fleeting moments of pleasure into lasting foundations for lifelong health, emotional fulfillment, and sustained happiness. Prioritizing sexual intimacy enriches relationships and offers profound and enduring physical, psychological and health benefits. By unleashing the erotic edge sexual intimacy provides a scientifically validated foundation for health and longevity.

CHAPTER 12

Mastering the Hormonal Clock: Discovering the Secrets to Aging Gracefully

"The afternoon knows what the morning never suspected."
—ROBERT FROST

Aging is akin to a delicate dance, choreographed by intricate shifts in our hormonal balance. These invisible chemical messengers govern nearly every facet of our lives—from metabolism and cognitive sharpness to immune strength and emotional resilience. Although hormonal decline naturally accompanies aging, its consequences aren't set in stone. By understanding these changes, making conscious lifestyle choices, and embracing targeted medical interventions, we can positively influence our health trajectory.

Insulin, the hormone acting as the body's diligent traffic controller, directs blood sugar efficiently into cells to fuel vitality and energy. In youth, insulin performs seamlessly, maintaining robust metabolism. However, with advancing age, cells often resist insulin's signals—much like a traffic jam forming on a once smoothly operating highway. This resistance triggers chronic inflammation, fat accumulation, and elevates the risk of metabolic disorders like type 2 diabetes. Incorporating resistance training and adopting a diet rich in fiber and low in refined sugars helps preserve insulin sensitivity, sustaining metabolic stability into later years.

Cortisol, often dubbed the "stress hormone," serves as both protector and potential adversary. Think of cortisol as the body's alarm system, sharpening focus and rapidly mobilizing energy to help you react swiftly in acute stress—such as narrowly avoiding an accident. Chronic stress, however, keeps this alarm persistently ringing, causing prolonged high cortisol levels. Over time, this persistent activation fuels inflammation, impairs cognitive function, and encourages harmful visceral fat accumulation.

Thyroid hormones, particularly T3 and T4, serve as the body's metabolic thermostat, governing energy levels, weight, temperature, and cognitive clarity. Think of them as skilled regulators, fine-tuning the pace of internal biological processes. With age, declining hormone levels slow metabolism, causing fatigue, sluggish digestion, and cognitive fog. Incorporating foods rich in iodine, selenium, and omega-3 fatty acids supports these essential regulators, maintaining metabolic balance and sustained well-being.

Growth hormone (GH), crucial for tissue repair, muscle preservation, and efficient fat metabolism, functions like a dedicated maintenance crew, tirelessly regenerating skin, muscle, and bone tissues. Natural GH production diminishes with age, causing decreased muscle mass, increased body fat, and slower recovery from injuries or exercise. Simple, sustainable lifestyle adjustments—such as regular strength training, quality sleep, and intermittent fasting—naturally boost your body's GH production, offering a safer path toward sustained health.

Testosterone, significant for both men and women, powerfully influences libido, muscle strength, bone density, and emotional well-being. Declining testosterone levels—known as andropause in men and contributing to menopause symptoms in women—can lead to fatigue, mood swings, and reduced vitality. Testosterone responds positively to strength training, stress management, and adequate sleep. Nutrients such as zinc and vitamin D provide additional support, while hormone replacement therapy remains effective for those facing severe deficiencies.

Estrogen plays a vital role in maintaining bone density, cardiovascular health, and cognitive sharpness. For women, the abrupt estrogen drop during menopause significantly increases the risk of osteoporosis, heart disease, and memory loss. Strength training, consuming phytoestrogen-rich foods like flaxseeds and soy, and adequate vitamin D intake help counteract these declines. Bioidentical hormone therapy offers further support for women experiencing challenging symptoms. Interestingly, estrogen is also important for men in smaller amounts derived from testosterone conversion, underscoring its broad importance across both sexes.

DHEA (dehydroepiandrosterone), an essential precursor to hormones like testosterone and estrogen. It strengthens immune function, boosts energy levels, and enhances stress resilience. Over time, however, DHEA levels naturally decline, like the gradual fading of daylight at sunset, correlating with increased inflammation and diminished vitality. Healthy lifestyle practices such as regular exercise, stress-reduction techniques, and nutrient-rich diets provide a strong foundation for naturally sustaining optimal DHEA levels.

Melatonin acts as a critical signaling molecule that aligns the body's circadian rhythms with environmental cues, particularly darkness. By synchronizing these rhythms, melatonin promotes restorative sleep, supports cellular repair, and regulates the timing of numerous biological pathways. Unfortunately, melatonin production declines with age, often resulting in restless nights, impaired immunity, and increased oxidative stress. Strategies for preserving melatonin include minimizing evening blue-light exposure—much like dimming lights before a theater performance—as well as maintaining consistent sleep schedules and designing tranquil sleep environments. When sleep difficulties persist, supplementation with melatonin may provide effective support.

Each hormone operates within an interconnected system, impacting not just how long we live but the richness and vitality of our years.

Hormonal decline is an inevitable aspect of aging, yet it remains within our influence. By comprehending hormones' profound roles, we empower ourselves to proactively intervene through mindful movement, nourishing nutrition, deliberate mindfulness practices, and targeted therapies—ensuring that the aging process remains marked by physical resilience, mental sharpness, and sustained energy.

Nutrition as the Foundation of Hormonal Balance

Our dietary choices provide the raw materials essential for hormone production, shaping everything from metabolism to emotional resilience. Omega-3 fatty acids—abundant in fatty fish, flaxseeds, and walnuts—act as internal firefighters, calming inflammation while simultaneously supporting cortisol balance and reproductive hormone synthesis. Zinc, found in shellfish, pumpkin seeds, and legumes, provides crucial fuel for testosterone production and immune strength. Magnesium, prevalent in leafy greens, nuts, and whole grains, stabilizes adrenal function, aiding cortisol management. Selenium, sourced from Brazil nuts, eggs, and seafood, quietly ensures optimal thyroid function. Beyond individual nutrients, stable blood sugar levels form the cornerstone of hormonal equilibrium. Reducing refined sugars and processed foods enhances insulin sensitivity, decreasing metabolic disruption risk. A fiber-rich diet filled with colorful, phytonutrient-dense fruits, vegetables, and whole grains nurtures gut health, further supporting balanced hormone regulation.

The Role of Exercise in Hormonal Optimization

Movement has a major influence on hormonal balance, enhancing insulin efficiency and reproductive vitality. Resistance training—through weights or bodyweight exercises—acts as a stimulus, elevating testosterone and growth hormone, essential for maintaining muscle mass, facilitating tissue repair, and boosting metabolic health. Cardiovascular activities like running, cycling, or swimming recalibrate insulin sensitivity and regulate cortisol by reducing visceral fat and increasing stress resilience. Moderation remains vital. Overtraining without adequate rest can elevate cortisol excessively, undermining exercise's hormonal benefits. A balanced approach combining resistance training, aerobic workouts, and flexibility practices such as yoga or Pilates offers a sustainable strategy for lifelong hormonal health.

The Essential Role of Sleep in Hormonal Regulation

Deep, restorative sleep is fundamental to hormonal well-being. During restful sleep, the body releases growth hormone—like a night crew diligently performing maintenance—facilitating tissue repair, muscle recovery, and effective fat metabolism. Melatonin, the sleep-inducing hormone, preserves circadian rhythms, fortifies immune responses, and reduces oxidative stress. Conversely, insufficient sleep prolongs elevated cortisol, disrupts insulin regulation, and interferes with appetite hormones such as leptin and ghrelin, causing increased cravings, sluggish metabolism, and unwanted weight gain. Prioritizing restful sleep through regular bedtime routines, reduced evening blue-light exposure, and tranquil sleep environments profoundly benefits overall hormonal harmony.

Managing Stress to Prevent Hormonal Disruptions

Chronic stress acts like an unwelcome guest overstaying their welcome, consistently disturbing hormonal harmony through prolonged cortisol elevation. While short-term cortisol spikes are crucial chronic elevations can significantly impair metabolism, immunity, and emotional stability. Mindfulness, meditation, yoga, and breathwork provide calming anchors, restoring balance within the nervous system. Additionally, embracing fulfilling activities such as tranquil nature walks, creative arts, or practicing gratitude can effectively offset stress-induced hormonal disruptions, bolstering emotional resilience.

Intermittent Fasting as a Metabolic and Hormonal Tool

Intermittent fasting offers a structured way to enhance metabolic and hormonal health, akin to periodically rebooting a computer for better efficiency. The widely practiced 16:8 protocol—fasting for 16 hours followed by an 8-hour eating window—supports insulin sensitivity, reduces inflammation, and boosts growth hormone production. However, intermittent fasting does not suit everyone. Those with adrenal fatigue or heightened hormonal sensitivities may experience added stress instead of benefits. Just as tailoring clothing ensures the right fit, fasting approaches should be adjusted based on personal stress levels, physical activity, and overall health to ensure that the practice remains beneficial rather than disruptive.

Targeted Supplementation for Hormonal Support

When thoughtfully chosen, supplementation can serve as a valuable tool in supporting hormonal health—akin to adding just the right seasoning to enhance a meal. Ashwagandha, an adaptogen, aids in cortisol regulation and enhances stress resilience. Maca root, celebrated for its potential to boost libido and energy, may also help balance reproductive hormones. Omega-3 fatty acids, available through fish oil or algae-based supplements, reduce inflammation and support cardiovascular health, indirectly stabilizing hormone levels. Vitamin D, essential for hormone synthesis, immune function, and mood regulation, is often deficient in those with limited sunlight exposure, making supplementation particularly beneficial. Consulting a healthcare provider ensures safe and effective incorporation of these targeted supplements.

Hormone Replacement Therapy: Restoring Balance When Necessary

For those experiencing substantial hormonal declines related to aging or particular medical conditions, hormone replacement therapy (HRT) provides an essential approach to restoring physiological balance and enhancing quality of life. In the next chapter, we'll take a closer look at hormone replacement therapy, offering deeper insights to guide informed decisions and optimize the benefits of this therapeutic approach.

Emerging Therapies and Future Directions in Hormonal Health

Scientific breakthroughs are rapidly transforming our understanding of hormonal health, paving the way for interventions that enhance hormone function, slow aging, and extend healthspan. Imagine these advances as bridges between today's realities and tomorrow's possibilities, allowing us to navigate aging with greater vitality. From peptide therapies designed to stimulate natural hormone production to groundbreaking gene-editing technologies, the future holds remarkable promise. At the same time, wearable technologies are evolving to provide real-time insights into metabolic function, stress levels, and hormonal fluctuations, enabling personalized interventions tailored to individual needs.

Peptide therapies stand among the most promising innovations, acting as short chains of amino acids that instruct the body to regulate its own hormone production. Unlike traditional hormone replacement, which introduces synthetic hormones, peptides synchronize with the body's natural rhythms. For instance, sermorelin stimulates the pituitary gland to produce growth hormone, supporting muscle health, tissue regeneration, and efficient fat metabolism. Other peptides, including CJC-1295 and Ipamorelin, show promise in reversing age-related declines in recovery, energy levels, and metabolic efficiency. By leveraging the body's own regulatory systems, peptide therapies offer a safer and more adaptive alternative to conventional hormone treatments.

Gene therapy is another transformative frontier poised to reshape endocrine aging. Advanced gene-editing tools such as CRISPR-Cas9 allow scientists to modify genes that influence hormone production, insulin sensitivity, and stress resilience—like carefully rewriting lines of code in the body's biological software. Researchers are exploring ways to enhance genes that promote growth hormone synthesis while silencing those that drive hormonal decline. In the future, gene therapy might directly introduce beneficial hormone-producing genes into tissues, creating long-term solutions for hormonal imbalances. Though still in experimental stages, the ability to delay or even reverse aging through targeted genetic modifications is an exciting and rapidly evolving field.

Beyond biological innovations, wearable technologies are reshaping how we monitor and manage hormonal health. Continuous glucose monitors (CGMs) provide real-time insights into insulin sensitivity, much like traffic updates helping you navigate congestion. Heart rate variability (HRV) trackers offer windows into stress and cortisol levels, while sleep-monitoring devices detect disruptions in melatonin production, offering guidance on improving sleep and recovery. The next generation of wearables may go even further, measuring hormones such as cortisol, estrogen, and testosterone through sweat or saliva. Coupled with AI-powered analytics, these devices could offer precise, personalized recommendations, bridging everyday health monitoring with advanced medical insights.

The convergence of these advanced therapies and technologies marks a transition from reactive treatments to proactive, personalized healthcare. Instead of addressing hormonal imbalances after symptoms arise, future interventions may prevent disruptions altogether, preserving health and vitality well before issues develop.

However, along with innovation come ethical and practical challenges. The long-term effects of gene editing and peptide treatments require further study, and ensuring equitable access to these advancements is critical. Additionally, the potential risks associated with unregulated use call for careful oversight and clear ethical guidelines. By emphasizing responsible development, rigorous research, and broad accessibility, these breakthroughs can benefit humanity safely and effectively.

The road ahead is inspiring. Gene editing, advanced wearable technologies, and other groundbreaking innovations continue to expand our horizons, redefining possibilities in hormonal health and longevity. With ongoing research and oversight, today's visionary science may soon become an integral part of daily health management, fundamentally transforming our experience of aging.

Hormonal Balance and the Science of Aging Well

Hormones serve as silent architects of aging, shaping our energy levels, metabolism, cognitive function, and emotional resilience. While hormonal decline is often seen as an inevitable aspect of growing older, it does not mean we must passively accept it. Armed with knowledge and proactive strategies, we can influence how we age—not just extending lifespan, but enhancing each year with energy, clarity, and resilience.

True hormonal balance goes beyond managing symptoms—it sustains well-being by preserving movement, mental sharpness, and overall fortitude. Nutrition, exercise, quality sleep, and stress management collectively support this balance, allowing the body to function optimally. Emerging scientific advancements further expand our options: bioidentical hormone therapies and personalized interventions offer innovative tools to address aging's biological shifts. These developments empower us to maintain long-term health and adaptability.

Hormones are not just chemical messengers; they are the undercurrent of how we move through the world—how we wake, how we focus, how we respond, how we recover. When balanced, they orchestrate a quiet, often invisible harmony that sustains both energy and ease. Disruption, however, is rarely inconspicuous. It can cloud thought, blunt motivation, and make even simple routines feel like resistance. To support hormonal health is not to defy age, but to remain in active dialogue with the body's shifting needs. And in doing so, we preserve not just function, but the capacity to remain curious, capable, and fully present as life unfolds.

CHAPTER 13

Hormone Replacement Therapy: Restoring Balance for Optimal Healthspan

"The body is like a piano, and happiness is like music. It is needful to have the instrument in good order."
—HENRY WARD BEECHER

Aging brings inevitable transformations, many of which stem from the gradual decline in hormone levels. These hormonal changes affect metabolism, cognition, and overall vitality. While aging is inevitable, hormone replacement therapy (HRT) offers a way to restore energy, support physiological balance, and extend healthspan.

This chapter presents an evidence-based exploration of hormone replacement therapy (HRT) and its role in supporting healthy aging. It outlines the potential benefits, known risks, and practical considerations, equipping readers to make informed decisions about its use. While often associated with symptom relief, HRT may also help preserve muscle strength, support cognitive function, and lower the risk of age-related conditions. When implemented with care, it offers the possibility of extending not just lifespan but also the period of life lived with physical capability and mental clarity—factors essential to maintaining quality of life in later years.

Understanding Hormone Replacement Therapy

Hormone replacement therapy (HRT) is a medical intervention designed to replenish declining hormone levels, alleviating symptoms associated with hormonal deficiencies. HRT helps mitigate age-related hormonal shifts, improving quality of life and lowering the risks of osteoporosis, cardiovascular disease, and cognitive decline. A personalized treatment approach ensures that HRT aligns with a person's unique health needs and goals.

HRT can be administered through several delivery methods, each offering distinct advantages depending on medical considerations and lifestyle preferences. Oral tablets provide convenience but may carry a slightly higher risk of blood clots due to liver metabolism. Transdermal patches and topical creams bypass the liver, ensuring steady hormone release while minimizing clotting risks. Subcutaneous pellets deliver extended-release therapy with fewer fluctuations, while injections, particularly for testosterone replacement, allow for controlled periodic dosing.

With proper medical supervision, HRT can be safely integrated into aging strategies, restoring hormonal balance and sustaining both mental and physical vitality over time. Continued advancements in research further refine its applications, solidifying HRT as a cornerstone of modern longevity medicine.

Hormone Replacement Therapy for Women: Tailoring Treatment for Optimal Health

For women navigating menopause and age-related hormonal shifts, hormone replacement therapy (HRT) serves as a tool for maintaining balance and well-being. While estrogen, progesterone, and testosterone form the foundation of most therapies, a truly comprehensive approach addresses the broader spectrum of hormonal interactions. Each hormone functions as part of a complex biological network, and carefully coordinating their roles can alleviate symptoms, improve quality of life, and reduce the risk of age-related diseases.

Estrogen Replacement Therapy (ERT) is often the primary treatment for menopausal symptoms such as hot flashes, night sweats, vaginal dryness, and mood fluctuations. Yet, estrogen's role extends beyond symptom relief—it is a key factor in bone health and cardiovascular function. Research indicates that initiating estrogen therapy within the first decade after menopause offers substantial benefits, including slowing bone loss and potentially reducing cognitive decline. However, maintaining balance is essential. After menopause, the body produces more estrone (E1), and excessive levels may elevate the risk of estrogen-sensitive conditions. Bioidentical estradiol (E2), which closely mimics natural estrogen, is commonly preferred for its compatibility with the body's biology. Women with a uterus typically combine estrogen with progesterone to prevent endometrial overgrowth and lower the risk of uterine cancer. Beyond this protective role, progesterone often enhances sleep quality and stabilizes mood, with exciting new research hinting that it may even help protect brain health. Larger studies will help illuminate how widely and consistently these promising benefits extend.

Testosterone, though often linked to men's health, is equally vital for women. It influences libido, mood, muscle strength, and cognitive function. Testosterone levels gradually decline after age 30, decreasing further during menopause and contributing to fatigue, diminished sexual desire, and loss of muscle tone. Available in gels, creams, or subcutaneous pellets, testosterone therapy can help restore energy, elevate mood, and maintain muscle and bone health. However, careful dosing is essential to prevent unwanted effects such as acne, excess hair growth, or voice changes. Similarly, DHEA (dehydroepiandrosterone), a precursor hormone for estrogen and testosterone, plays a significant role in energy regulation, stress resilience, and immune function. As levels decline with age, some women experience fatigue, emotional instability, and increased susceptibility to illness. Low-dose supplementation may help restore vitality, though careful monitoring is required to avoid androgenic side effects.

Intrarosa offers an additional, targeted option for women experiencing discomfort from vaginal dryness and sensitivity post-menopause. Containing prasterone (DHEA), Intrarosa converts within the body into natural hormones, revitalizing vaginal moisture, elasticity, and overall tissue health. This approach effectively alleviates discomfort, promoting physical ease during intimacy and supporting emotional closeness. Intrarosa provides a reassuring alternative to traditional estrogen-based treatments, delivering relief while minimizing common concerns associated with estrogen therapies, thereby empowering women to comfortably reconnect in their relationships.

A Holistic Approach to Women's Hormonal Health

Hormone replacement therapy (HRT) offers valuable relief from the symptoms of hormonal decline, yet achieving true hormonal balance is much like cultivating a flourishing garden—it requires attentive care from multiple angles. Lifestyle interventions can enrich hormonal health. For instance, incorporating regular strength training into one's life can serve as steady fuel for testosterone production, supporting both physical vitality and emotional resilience. Similarly, embracing a nutrient-rich diet can nourish the thyroid and optimize insulin function. Foods abundant in colorful vegetables, healthy proteins, and essential fats lay a firm foundation for energy and metabolic harmony.

Deliberate practices such as meditation, controlled breathing, or even moments of stillness can help regulate cortisol—the body's primary stress hormone—easing tension and supporting physiological balance. These peaceful moments do more than manage stress—they amplify the effectiveness of hormone therapies, nurturing a harmonious environment for wellness. Regular hormonal monitoring complements these lifestyle practices. Guided by precise testing and individualized adjustments, this monitoring acts like a compass, reliably directing therapy to remain safe and effective over time.

For women seeking to restore and maintain their hormonal equilibrium, partnering closely with knowledgeable healthcare providers is essential. Together, they create personalized strategies carefully attuned to each woman's unique physiology, medical history, and personal lifestyle. Proactively addressing hormonal shifts—whether through bioidentical hormone therapy aligned to her natural chemistry, targeted supplementation, or lifestyle modifications—empowers each woman to view aging as a chapter filled with renewed strength and well-being.

Hormone Replacement Therapy for Men: Enhancing Vitality and Performance

As men age, shifts in hormonal balance can reshape their sense of vitality, mental sharpness, and overall wellness. Think of testosterone as the master regulator of a complex ecosystem, coordinating physical energy, mood, muscle strength, and cognitive clarity. Beginning as early as their 30s, men experience a gradual decline in testosterone, often leading to decreased energy, reduced libido, muscle loss, and subtle cognitive changes. While this decline is natural, it need not define a man's experience of aging. Hormone replacement therapy (HRT) provides precise support, effectively addressing hormonal deficiencies to promote sustained energy, emotional resilience, and overall quality of life.

Testosterone Replacement Therapy (TRT)

Among hormonal interventions for men, testosterone replacement therapy (TRT) stands out as one of the most widely studied and impactful. Specifically addressing symptoms of low testosterone—commonly known as andropause—TRT can effectively ease fatigue, enhance libido, reduce fat accumulation, and improve mood stability, thereby elevating overall quality of life.

In addition to enhancing physical and sexual vitality, TRT aids in muscle maintenance, fat metabolism, and cardiovascular health. Research highlights that maintaining optimal testosterone levels enhances insulin sensitivity, reducing the risk of metabolic conditions like type 2 diabetes. Additionally, testosterone plays a role in cognitive function, supporting memory, mental sharpness, and emotional stability. Emerging research even suggests that sustaining healthy testosterone levels may offer protection against neurodegenerative diseases such as Alzheimer's.

TRT is available in multiple forms, including transdermal gels, injections, patches, and subcutaneous pellets, each adaptable to individual needs. Regular monitoring ensures precise dosing, reducing potential risks such as elevated red blood cell counts or fluid retention. Previous concerns linking TRT to prostate cancer have largely been dispelled, with recent studies showing no significant risk when therapy is properly managed. In fact, balanced testosterone is now recognized as a contributor to prostate health and longevity.

For men seeking to regain strength and vitality, TRT stands as one of the most effective tools for enhancing both lifespan and well-being.

DHEA and Growth Hormone: Supporting Energy and Recovery

Testosterone does not act alone; it relies on a supportive network of hormones. Among these, DHEA (dehydroepiandrosterone) plays an important role as a precursor to testosterone and estrogen, supporting energy, immunity, and stress resilience. As DHEA levels decline with age, men may experience fatigue, reduced libido, and slower recovery from physical exertion. Like replenishing nutrient-rich soil, supplementing DHEA under medical supervision can help restore hormonal balance, bolster resilience, and reduce inflammation. However, careful monitoring is necessary to avoid unwanted side effects.

Growth hormone (GH), along with its key partner insulin-like growth factor 1 (IGF-1), plays a vital role in tissue repair, muscle health, and fat metabolism. GH continuously supports muscle regeneration and metabolic efficiency. Yet, as men age, natural GH production declines, leading to slower muscle recovery, increased fat accumulation, and diminished overall energy. While direct GH supplementation remains controversial due to potential side effects, peptide-based therapies such as sermorelin and CJC-1295 physiologically stimulate the body's own GH production, potentially offering a safer alternative. Lifestyle adjustments—including resistance training, high-intensity interval workouts, and quality sleep—further reinforce these therapies, strengthening muscle health and metabolic resilience.

Holistic Hormonal Health for Men: Personalized Strategies Beyond Therapy

Optimizing hormonal health requires a personalized approach that aligns with individual needs, medical history, and lifestyle preferences. While testosterone therapy remains a foundational pillar of male hormone replacement therapy (HRT), a truly comprehensive approach extends beyond TRT to incorporate other key hormones, including DHEA, growth hormone, thyroid hormones, and cortisol. Addressing these interconnected systems allows men to sustain peak performance, emotional resilience, and metabolic efficiency.

Advancements in precision medicine, wearable technologies, and real-time biomarker monitoring empower men with greater control over their hormonal health. These innovations act as navigational tools, offering real-time feedback on internal fluctuations and enabling proactive health adjustments. A data-driven approach allows for informed decisions, balancing safety with optimized therapeutic outcomes. Integrating targeted medical interventions with foundational lifestyle practices—such as strength training, nutrient-dense diets, restorative sleep, and mindful stress management—creates a robust framework for lasting health. Rather than viewing aging as inevitable decline, men can reframe this phase of life as an opportunity to cultivate resilience, self-assurance, and long-term vitality.

Bioidentical vs. Synthetic Hormones

All hormone replacement therapies aim to restore hormonal balance, but distinguishing between bioidentical and synthetic hormones is essential. Bioidentical hormones share the exact molecular structure of hormones naturally produced by the body, allowing them to interact seamlessly with hormone receptors. In contrast, synthetic hormones often have structural variations, potentially changing their biological effects. For example, conjugated equine estrogens (CEE), derived from the urine of pregnant mares, include multiple estrogenic compounds differing structurally from human estrogen. These differences can result in distinct physiological responses. Similarly, certain synthetic progestins, structurally unlike natural progesterone, have been linked in some studies to increased risks of adverse effects, including a higher likelihood of blood clots and breast cancer.

Often misunderstood, the distinction between bioidentical and synthetic hormones hinges specifically on their chemical structure—not their source or manufacturing process. A hormone derived from plant sources can still be synthetic if its molecular structure isn't an exact replica of human hormones. Conversely, hormones created entirely in laboratories can be considered bioidentical if they precisely match the molecular composition of naturally occurring human hormones.

FDA-Approved and Compounded Bioidentical Hormones

Bioidentical hormones come in two primary forms: FDA-approved formulations and compounded preparations. FDA-approved bioidentical hormones undergo rigorous evaluation to verify safety, efficacy, and quality. Manufactured under stringent regulatory standards, these products ensure consistent purity and accurate dosing. Estradiol patches, progesterone capsules, and testosterone gels are common examples, all thoroughly studied in clinical trials.

On the other hand, compounded bioidentical hormones are custom-formulated preparations individually prepared by compounding pharmacies to address specific patient needs. This customization offers flexibility in dosing and alternative delivery methods—such as creams, lozenges, or injections—but compounded formulations are not FDA-approved. Consequently, their lack of standardization raises valid concerns about variability in potency, purity, and effectiveness. Without large-scale clinical trials confirming their safety, major medical organizations, including the American College of Obstetricians and Gynecologists, caution against the routine use of compounded bioidentical hormones.

Common Myths About Hormone Replacement Therapy

Few health topics ignite as much discussion and confusion as hormone replacement therapy. One of the most persistent myths is the belief that HRT inevitably leads to cancer. This misconception largely stems from the early concerns raised by the Women's Health Initiative (WHI) study in 2002, which identified increased risks of breast cancer, stroke, and cardiovascular disease with certain synthetic hormone formulations—particularly conjugated equine estrogens (CEE) and synthetic progestins. However, subsequent research has refined these findings, showing that the risks associated with HRT depend heavily on factors like hormone type, dosage, administration method, and individual health status.

Bioidentical hormones, particularly estradiol and micronized progesterone, appear to carry lower risks compared to their synthetic counterparts. Additionally, estrogen therapy alone has not been linked to increased breast cancer risk for women who have undergone a hysterectomy. For those needing combined therapy, it is essential to consider personal health profiles, as the effects of progesterone on breast tissue vary significantly among formulations. Instead of being inherently dangerous, HRT's potential impact on cancer risk is influenced by genetics, overall health, and lifestyle. When prescribed carefully and monitored, hormone therapy can be a safe and effective tool for long-term well-being.

A common misconception is that hormone therapy only addresses severe menopause or andropause symptoms, ignoring its extensive additional benefits. While relief from hot flashes, night sweats, mood swings, and sleep disturbances is a key motivator, HRT offers many additional advantages that extend well beyond immediate symptom management. Estrogen therapy plays an essential role in maintaining bone density, reducing the risks of osteoporosis and fractures, and improving metabolic health by enhancing insulin sensitivity. Furthermore, research suggests that estrogen therapy initiated during the "critical window" following menopause may not only improve cognitive function but could also lower the risk of Alzheimer's disease.

Men experiencing declining testosterone levels can face gradual changes over time affecting energy, libido, muscle mass, and overall vitality—changes effectively managed through testosterone replacement therapy (TRT). While TRT is effective in restoring these functions, it should be prescribed only when medically necessary, as inappropriate use can lead to increased red blood cell production, prostate enlargement, and cardiovascular risks. When managed appropriately, TRT can slow the effects of hormonal aging and significantly enhance quality of life.

HRT is undergoing a transformative shift, driven by advances in precision medicine, genetic testing, and personalized treatment plans. By assessing biomarkers such as CYP19A1—an enzyme involved in estrogen production—and sex hormone-binding globulin (SHBG), a protein regulating hormone availability, healthcare providers can predict individual hormone metabolism more accurately. This personalized approach enables safer, more effective hormone treatments tailored precisely to each person's unique biology.

Innovative delivery methods are enhancing the effectiveness and ease of hormone replacement therapy, making treatments simpler and more comfortable than ever before. Transdermal estradiol patches, applied to the skin, provide a steady, continuous release of estrogen. Progesterone can be administered sublingually—comfortably dissolving beneath the tongue—to maintain stable and consistent hormone levels. Another convenient advancement is the use of long-acting testosterone implants: tiny pellets placed just beneath the skin that gradually release testosterone, minimizing hormone fluctuations and enhancing therapeutic outcomes. Additionally, exciting new peptide-based therapies such as CJC-1295 and sermorelin are emerging. These specialized peptides encourage the body's own natural production of growth hormone, thereby improving its capacity to heal tissues, recover from injuries, and regenerate more effectively. With such thoughtful innovations, hormone replacement therapy continues to evolve, offering greater hope and improved quality of life.

As the field of HRT continues to evolve, ongoing research will refine protocols, improve safety profiles, and make therapies more accessible. The future of hormone therapy holds great promise, offering powerful tools to improve healthspan and longevity while allowing each of us to approach aging with confidence and a sense of control.

The Path Forward: Maximizing Health Through Hormonal Balance

Aging is an inevitable journey, yet how we experience it is far from predetermined. Hormone replacement therapy (HRT) is not only a medical response to hormonal decline—it's a transformative path toward embracing life's later chapters with vitality, confidence, and emotional fortitude. As key hormones naturally decline, the body gradually undergoes changes that influence physical strength, energy levels, emotional balance, and mental clarity. These changes need not be passively accepted. Through thoughtful interventions, people can actively shape a journey marked by adaptability and purpose.

The true power of hormone therapy lies in its capacity to honor the unique experiences of each person. Aging unfolds differently for everyone, and personalized hormonal care recognizes and respects this complexity. Individualized HRT goes beyond symptom relief. It empowers people to approach their later years with renewed optimism, vigor, and possibility. For women, carefully timed estrogen therapy provides benefits that sustain physical and emotional well-being, nurturing not just health but the ability to thrive emotionally and socially. Men similarly benefit from carefully managed testosterone therapy, gaining renewed strength, energy, and a positive outlook toward life.

Beyond potentially just prolonging life, hormone therapy enriches its quality and depth. When combined with intentional lifestyle practices—mindful physical activity, wholesome nutrition, stress reduction, and restorative sleep—HRT becomes an essential component of a multidimensional approach to aging. This integrated strategy enhances personal resilience, emotional fulfillment, and meaningful engagement with life's many stages, turning aging into an era of personal growth, connection, and continued discovery.

Thanks to advancements in hormone therapy, expectations about aging are shifting significantly. Ongoing innovations continue to broaden these possibilities, reshaping how society understands and navigates the aging process. Modern hormone therapies do more than delay physical decline; they support a dynamic, purposeful approach to later life, fostering greater resilience, satisfaction, and well-being.

Choosing hormone therapy signifies a deliberate commitment to cultivating internal balance, laying the groundwork for fully embracing life's unfolding possibilities. With hormones properly balanced, aging becomes less constrained by physical limitations. Instead, it emerges as an opportunity-rich phase characterized by deeper connections, ongoing exploration, and continued personal growth.

PART III
Rewriting the Rules of Aging—Longevity Science and Biohacking

"The reasonable man adapts himself to the world; the unreasonable one persists in trying to adapt the world to himself. Therefore all progress depends on the unreasonable man."
—George Bernard Shaw

Biohacking often conjures images of bold self-experimentation, but longevity science encompasses a far richer and more systematic approach. It includes pioneering individual efforts alongside thorough scientific testing, regulatory oversight, and careful integration into conventional medical practice. As cutting-edge longevity treatments transition from experimental interventions to broader use, their potential public health impacts—and the ethical questions they raise—require thoughtful consideration. This section explores these real-world implications, highlighting how emerging therapies might fundamentally change our collective perception of aging.

Biohacking certainly remains an integral aspect of this growing discipline, offering dynamic tools that empower us to actively manage our health. Yet longevity science extends well beyond personal optimization alone. At its core, it prioritizes rigorously tested, evidence-based therapies that are emerging from advanced research and moving toward adoption in clinical settings. Clearly distinguishing between self-directed enhancement methods and scientifically validated interventions is essential for navigating this rapidly evolving landscape safely and effectively.

Much like pioneers venturing into uncharted territories, biohackers tread carefully between the promise of discovery and the uncertainties of experimentation. Self-testing can offer unique personal insights but also carries inherent risks, particularly when novel treatments lack extensive long-term safety data or standardized treatment protocols. Optimizing health should never come at the expense of well-being. Navigating this complex and swiftly changing terrain demands discernment, solid scientific knowledge, and collaboration with trusted medical and longevity experts. By balancing innovation with prudence, those aiming to extend their healthspan and lifespan can ensure their journey remains forward-looking, safe, responsible, and rooted in rigorous science.

CHAPTER 14

Rapamycin and Rapalogs: Pioneering the Anti-Aging Frontier

"The only way to discover the limits of the possible is to go beyond them into the impossible."
—ARTHUR C. CLARKE

Across centuries, humankind has pursued ways to delay, halt, or even reverse aging. Myths of mystical fountains and legendary elixirs have long captured the imagination, but rapamycin stands apart—not for folklore, but for the strength of its scientific promise. Originally used to prevent organ rejection in transplant recipients, rapamycin has since drawn widespread attention as one of the most consequential longevity discoveries in recent decades. Today, researchers are exploring its potential not only to extend lifespan, but also to expand healthspan—the years marked by vitality and freedom from chronic disease.

At the center of rapamycin's potential is its ability to influence a fundamental biological system: the mTOR pathway, which governs whether cells prioritize growth or restoration. By selectively inhibiting a key component known as mTOR Complex 1 (mTORC1), rapamycin shifts cellular activity toward repair. This change activates autophagy—the body's internal recycling mechanism—allowing cells to clear damaged components and maintain internal stability. The resulting cellular state closely mirrors that induced by caloric restriction, a well-documented intervention known to extend lifespan in multiple species. By reproducing these effects pharmacologically, rapamycin presents a promising longevity strategy rooted in the body's own restorative systems.

Clearing the Wreckage: Rapamycin's Role in Inflammaging, Senescence, and Metabolic Health

Building on its role in cellular repair, rapamycin also targets two major biological processes that accelerate aging: chronic inflammation and cellular senescence. As the immune system ages, it often shifts into a state of low-grade, persistent inflammation—a phenomenon known as *inflammaging*—which quietly drives conditions such as cardiovascular disease, neurodegeneration, and metabolic dysfunction. Rapamycin helps counter this process by lowering key biomarkers of inflammation and promoting immune balance in aging tissues.

Senescent cells—damaged cells that stop dividing but continue to release harmful signals—pose another threat. These so-called "zombie cells" linger in tissues, undermining nearby healthy cells and accelerating tissue degeneration. Rapamycin reduces both the burden of senescent cells and the damaging compounds they release, offering a precise intervention to mitigate tissue breakdown.

Its influence extends further. In muscle tissue, rapamycin supports the activity of satellite cells, which are essential for muscle repair, by maintaining autophagy and reducing stress. This may help preserve strength, mobility, and independence as we age. In metabolic systems, it enhances energy flexibility—allowing the body to shift more efficiently between glucose and fat use—while improving insulin sensitivity and liver function. Animal studies have further shown that rapamycin influences liver gene expression in ways associated with enhanced metabolic adaptation and resilience. As human trials continue, rapamycin remains one of the most promising tools in the evolving landscape of longevity science.

Revitalizing Immune Function and Protecting Cognitive Health

Immune systems naturally weaken over time, leaving older adults increasingly vulnerable to infections and with reduced vaccine responsiveness. Rapamycin stimulates immune responsiveness, effectively revitalizing an aging immune system. Clinical trials suggest older adults receiving rapamycin experience heightened vaccine effectiveness and fewer infections, offering substantial implications for improved immune resilience.

Rapamycin's protective benefits also extend into the intricate neural networks of the brain. With age, harmful proteins—such as amyloid-beta and tau—accumulate, contributing to Alzheimer's and Parkinson's diseases. Rapamycin activates autophagy, facilitating the clearance of these damaging protein accumulations, preserving neural integrity. Animal studies have revealed improved memory, reduced brain inflammation, and healthier neural pathways in rapamycin-treated mice. Human studies currently underway will be crucial in determining the full scope of these immune system and neurological benefits.

Insights from Animal Studies: Longevity Extended by Rapamycin

Consistent animal studies confirm rapamycin's extraordinary power to prolong lifespan. In mice, median and maximum lifespans typically increase by 20–30%. Remarkably, these gains occur even when treatment begins later in life. Rapamycin doesn't only delay aging; it appears capable of reversing certain age-related declines, demonstrating impressive versatility. Yet, extending such findings to humans demands caution. Larger, long-term human trials remain essential to confidently establish rapamycin's ability to boost human healthspan and lifespan. Still, lifespan-extending effects appear consistently across a remarkable variety of species—from yeast and worms to fruit flies—highlighting rapamycin's significant impact on evolutionarily conserved biological mechanisms. Although the complexity of human biology introduces uncertainties, this broad cross-species efficacy positions rapamycin as an exceptionally promising candidate within longevity science.

Current Human Protocols—Off-Label Use of Rapamycin for Longevity and Healthspan

The off-label use of rapamycin to enhance longevity and healthspan has increasingly attracted scientific and public attention. Initially approved by the FDA to prevent kidney transplant rejection and manage certain medical conditions, rapamycin has remarkably transitioned into a promising longevity intervention. Contemporary protocols differ significantly from traditional daily, high-dose immunosuppressive regimens, emphasizing instead carefully timed, intermittent dosing schedules. By briefly pausing mTOR complex 1 (mTORC1)—similar to temporarily halting activity on a busy production line—these intervals facilitate cellular repair, reduce inflammation, and improve metabolic function.

Several dosing methods have emerged from comprehensive animal studies, clinical observations, and ongoing human trials. One popular protocol involves administering weekly oral doses ranging from 3 to 10 mg, selectively inhibiting mTORC1 activity. This targeted inhibition achieves therapeutic benefits while minimizing chronic suppression of mTOR complex 2 (mTORC2), thus reducing metabolic risks. Another strategy, intermittent pulse dosing, employs higher doses (5 to 15 mg) taken every 10 to 14 days. This approach mirrors the effects observed with intermittent fasting or caloric restriction, briefly allowing mTOR activity to rebound. Despite its conceptual promise, robust human data supporting pulse dosing remains limited. Alternatively, daily low-dose rapamycin (1 to 2 mg), adapted from practices in transplant medicine and oncology, offers continuous mild mTOR suppression but carries greater potential for adverse effects, necessitating careful consideration.

Combination therapies pairing rapamycin with agents like metformin or acarbose are also under investigation. Animal studies, especially those conducted by the National Institute on Aging's Interventions Testing

Program (ITP), suggest these combinations could offer synergistic longevity benefits. However, the complexity and increased risk of drug interactions associated with combination therapies necessitate cautious exploration in human populations.

Clinicians typically begin rapamycin therapy conservatively, around 1 to 2 mg weekly, adjusting dosages based on patient responses. Dose adjustments rely on monitoring protocols detailed in the subsequent section. Ultimately, rapamycin serves as a promising but experimental component within a personalized health and longevity framework.

Potential Risks and Safety Considerations

While rapamycin represents a compelling advancement in longevity science, careful management is essential to balance its potential benefits against known risks. Ongoing vigilance through regular monitoring facilitates prompt identification and mitigation of possible adverse effects.

Commonly reported side effects include transient mouth ulcers, generally mild and responsive to dosage adjustments or supportive care. Lipid metabolism may also be affected, occasionally leading to increased cholesterol or triglyceride levels. Routine lipid screenings allow early detection, enabling effective management through lifestyle modifications or medications such as statins.

Intermittent dosing typically preserves or improves immune function compared to continuous, high-dose treatment. Nevertheless, timing is critical; temporarily suspending rapamycin during acute infections or immediately post-surgery—periods requiring robust immune responses—is advisable. Initial gastrointestinal disturbances (nausea, diarrhea, mild abdominal discomfort) or transient fatigue may occur when therapy begins, typically resolving quickly as the body adjusts or following minor dosage refinements.

Effective rapamycin treatment requires comprehensive baseline assessments, including evaluations of lipid profiles, liver function, complete blood counts, fasting insulin and glucose levels, rapamycin trough concentrations, inflammatory markers, and immune cell subsets. Regular follow-up assessments ensure sustained safety and therapeutic effectiveness.

Incorporating rapamycin into broader lifestyle practices—such as balanced nutrition, consistent physical activity, and stress management—further enhances its efficacy and reduces potential risks. Although short-term studies in humans have yielded promising results, long-term implications of intermittent rapamycin use remain uncertain. Until extensive long-term data become available, cautious and professionally supervised application ensures the substantial promise of rapamycin continues to outweigh associated risks.

Rapamycin's Path Forward: Future Human Trials and Research Directions

The future trajectory of rapamycin research is exceptionally promising, opening compelling avenues within longevity science and preventive medicine. Researchers continually refine rapamycin's therapeutic capabilities, striving to maximize its benefits and reduce adverse outcomes. Notably, the development of rapalogs—compounds structurally related to rapamycin yet engineered for improved safety and tolerability—represents significant progress toward precision medicine. These agents offer potential enhancements in metabolic health, targeted physiological protection, and sustainable management of aging-related conditions.

Another major research focus targets age-associated frailty, characterized by declining muscle strength, mobility, and overall resilience. Current clinical studies are examining whether combining intermittent low-dose rapamycin with resistance training effectively preserves muscle strength, endurance, and independence. Positive outcomes could establish rapamycin firmly as an essential therapeutic tool for maintaining quality of life among aging populations.

Emerging research specifically aims to bolster immune resilience through refined dosing strategies, potentially improving vaccine responsiveness and infection resistance. Such targeted investigations could elevate rapamycin to a critical immunomodulatory role, substantially extending healthspan.

Clarifying long-term efficacy and safety through extensive human trials remains a crucial objective. While animal studies consistently demonstrate lifespan extension, robust human evidence remains limited. Upcoming trials aim to elucidate rapamycin's long-term effects on cardiovascular health, neuroprotection, and metabolic regulation. Researchers are particularly enthusiastic about novel combination therapies, such as pairing rapamycin with senolytics, possibly amplifying anti-aging benefits through complementary mechanisms.

As scientific understanding expands, rapamycin may transition from an experimental intervention to a cornerstone of preventive medicine. Although explicit regulatory approval for anti-aging remains aspirational, current advancements strongly suggest rapamycin's future significance in enhancing healthspan.

Rapamycin is not a universal cure, yet its promise signals a profound shift in how society approaches aging. Can we meaningfully reshape the biological trajectory of aging? Ongoing rapamycin research may soon yield definitive insights.

The Rise of Rapalogs in Longevity Science

Building on the remarkable achievements of rapamycin, researchers have begun developing rapalogs—modified compounds designed to refine therapeutic potential and overcome some of rapamycin's clinical limitations. Although rapamycin's ability to influence aging biology is firmly established, its clinical application has faced challenges, such as immune suppression, unpredictable pharmacokinetics, and complicated dosing regimens. Rapalogs represent a more sophisticated evolution, offering enhanced precision, bioavailability, and safety, thereby advancing the field of longevity therapies.

Rapalogs specifically target the same longevity-promoting pathways as rapamycin—primarily mTORC1—but structural adjustments provide more predictable dosing and minimize immune-related risks. Compounds like everolimus and ridaforolimus, already clinically approved for cancer treatment and immune modulation, are now undergoing exploration for broader applications. Researchers are particularly interested in their potential to enhance metabolic health, immune resilience, and neuroprotection in aging populations. Through targeted and sustained modulation of mTOR, rapalogs significantly advance personalized longevity medicine.

Expanding the Potential of mTOR Modulation

Rapalogs maintain rapamycin's core biological functions, such as activating autophagy, regulating cellular metabolism, and suppressing inflammation, but they bring refined pharmacological characteristics to the table. This careful balance between effective mTOR inhibition and preservation of immune function increases their viability for long-term therapeutic use.

Unlike rapamycin, which frequently requires precise dosing adjustments, rapalogs offer greater flexibility, substantially reducing immune suppression risks. This advantage is particularly valuable in longevity-focused treatments, where maintaining robust immune function alongside managing cellular aging is essential.

Each rapalog demonstrates unique, tissue-specific effects that enhance targeted clinical applications. For instance, everolimus shows promise in boosting vaccine responses among older adults, potentially mitigating immune senescence. Rapalogs like ridaforolimus, with shorter half-lives, facilitate intermittent mTORC1 suppression followed by adequate recovery intervals. Such intermittent dosing strategies may reproduce caloric restriction benefits without sustained suppression.

Moreover, rapalogs may significantly contribute to neuroprotection and metabolic health. By modulating neuronal autophagy and reducing neuroinflammation, their selective inhibition of mTORC1 could enhance insulin sensitivity and lipid metabolism, potentially avoiding metabolic compromises sometimes seen with chronic rapamycin use.

Potential Synergies: Combining Rapalogs with Other Longevity Interventions

When thoughtfully combined with complementary interventions, rapalogs could offer more substantial longevity benefits than single-agent use. Just as an orchestra achieves harmony through diverse instruments playing together, integrating rapalogs with senolytics like dasatinib and quercetin may enhance tissue regeneration by effectively removing senescent cells. This approach resembles clearing a garden of debris to allow new growth.

Another promising strategy pairs rapalogs with caloric restriction mimetics such as metformin or resveratrol, compounds known to activate complementary biological pathways (AMPK and sirtuins). The combined therapies may create a balanced metabolic environment that mitigates potential risks from sustained mTOR inhibition. Adding NAD+ precursors, like NMN or NR, could further support mitochondrial vitality and cellular repair, amplifying the rejuvenating impact of rapalogs.

Challenges and Considerations: Safety, Risks, and Unanswered Questions

While rapalogs offer significant promise, their responsible use demands careful dosing and awareness of potential risks. Picture rapalogs as precise medical tools, powerful yet requiring skilled handling for optimal safety and effectiveness. Although rapalogs generally exhibit improved safety profiles compared to rapamycin, concerns persist about their long-term metabolic effects. For example, prolonged mTORC1 inhibition might inadvertently impact mTORC2—a critical pathway in glucose metabolism and insulin signaling—raising potential issues regarding insulin resistance distinct from lipid metabolism concerns seen with rapamycin.

Future research needs to clarify rapalogs' impacts on specific tissues reliant on mTOR activity, such as muscles and connective tissue. Continuous mTORC1 suppression could potentially impair muscle recovery, slow wound healing, or weaken adaptive immune responses. Strategies such as intermittent dosing or combined supportive therapies might mitigate these risks.

Additionally, prolonged rapalog use could lead to diminishing returns, as persistent mTORC1 inhibition might provoke compensatory biological adaptations, gradually reducing effectiveness. Researchers are actively investigating solutions, including periodic dosing breaks or combination therapies, to maintain sustained efficacy.

For safety monitoring guidelines—including baseline assessments and regular follow-ups—please consult previously detailed recommendations for rapamycin. As additional rapalog-specific research emerges, optimal dosing protocols will be refined, fully unlocking their potential within longevity medicine.

The Future: Rapamycin, Rapalogs, and the Dawn of Age-Modifying Medicine

Rapamycin and its derivatives, the rapalogs, represent a remarkable turning point in longevity science. Initially developed as immunosuppressants, these compounds have evolved into pioneering agents that influence fundamental processes of aging. The scientific evidence supporting rapamycin's potential is compelling. It helps preserve muscle strength, boosts metabolic resilience, and reduces chronic inflammation. Rapamycin even rejuvenates immune responses and offers valuable neuroprotective benefits. Consistent animal studies reinforce its lifespan-extending capabilities, providing substantial grounds for optimism.

Yet important questions remain. Considerable clinical research is still needed to determine rapamycin's safety, optimal dosage, appropriate duration of treatment, and long-term efficacy in humans. Researchers continue to explore potential long-term safety concerns associated with sustained use. Side effects might vary at different ages. Additionally, interactions with medications or supplements commonly used by older adults need careful investigation.

As longevity science advances toward precision medicine, rapamycin and rapalogs offer promising avenues for personalized therapies. By tailoring regimens to individual genetic profiles, existing health conditions, and biomarker assessments, benefits can be optimized and risks minimized. C Thoughtful exploration of rapamycin's therapeutic potential could significantly reshape humanity's relationship with aging. Yet critical questions remain: How might extended healthspan alter the ways we set goals, pursue ambitions, and define the stages and milestones of our lives? What ethical frameworks will ensure equitable access to these powerful interventions? And is society prepared—economically, socially, and philosophically—for a future in which the consequences of aging are substantially delayed, even as aging itself remains inevitable?

CHAPTER 15

Metformin: Reimagining a Diabetes Drug for Longevity

"Discovery consists of seeing what everybody has seen and thinking what nobody has thought."
—ALBERT SZENT-GYORGI

For decades, metformin has reliably served as a trusted medication for type 2 diabetes, praised for its effectiveness in regulating blood sugar. Recently, however, this humble drug has captured scientific attention for an entirely different—and remarkable—reason: its potential to slow the fundamental process of aging. Growing evidence suggests metformin influences critical biological pathways related to longevity, indicating it might help people not just live longer but also enjoy healthier, more vibrant lives.

Unlike many experimental anti-aging treatments, metformin is already widely available, affordable, and extensively studied in humans. Its advantages seem to extend far beyond glucose control, touching processes as diverse as metabolism, cellular repair, inflammation, and even gene expression. Think of metformin as medicine's Swiss Army knife—widely accessible, practical, and surprisingly versatile, possibly holding keys to healthier aging hidden within its familiar form. Yet, despite these exciting possibilities, current evidence remains observational—demonstrating intriguing connections but stopping short of proving causation. This leaves a crucial question unanswered: can metformin genuinely slow human aging, or are its apparent benefits merely a fortunate byproduct of improved metabolic health?

Unlocking Longevity Pathways: How Metformin Works

At the cellular level, aging is a complex interplay of metabolic shifts, chronic inflammation, and accumulated damage. Remarkably, metformin appears to target several of these crucial processes simultaneously. One of its significant effects involves activating AMP-activated protein kinase (AMPK), often depicted as a "metabolic switch." Picture AMPK as a diligent manager, carefully adjusting energy usage within cells during stressful times. By stimulating AMPK, metformin enhances mitochondrial performance, stabilizes glucose metabolism, and boosts insulin sensitivity, mimicking beneficial effects seen with caloric restriction—a well-established longevity strategy in animal studies.

Metformin's influence, however, extends beyond metabolism. It also modulates the mechanistic Target of Rapamycin (mTOR) pathway, a central coordinator of cellular growth and repair. Imagine mTOR as an energetic supervisor, constantly directing construction and expansion. Metformin encourages this supervisor to pause, granting cells vital time for cleanup. By reducing mTOR activity, metformin promotes autophagy, the cellular housekeeping mechanism that clears away damaged proteins and worn-out organelles. This cleanup is essential for preventing molecular debris buildup, reducing tissue deterioration, and protecting against age-related diseases.

Aging involves more than just declining metabolism. Chronic inflammation, commonly called "inflammaging," quietly fuels heart disease, neurodegeneration, and metabolic dysfunction over time. Metformin helps counteract this damaging cycle by inhibiting a critical inflammatory pathway known as NF-κB. Additionally, it fosters a healthier gut microbiome—the bustling community of beneficial bacteria in our digestive tract—that profoundly influences immune health and metabolic stability.

Intriguingly, recent research suggests metformin might even influence genetic mechanisms, such as DNA methylation—an essential epigenetic process controlling gene expression across a lifespan. Although this research area is still developing, the possibility that metformin can slow genetic hallmarks of aging adds another exciting dimension to its potential as a longevity-enhancing drug.

Taken together, these diverse mechanisms form a compelling narrative: metformin addresses multiple aging pathways simultaneously, from metabolism and inflammation to cellular repair and potentially genetic regulation. However, the fundamental question persists—will these cellular and molecular effects translate into tangible longevity benefits for humans?

Insights from Animal and Human Studies

Across various species, from tiny worms to mammals, metformin consistently links to extended lifespans and delayed age-related decline. For instance, mice treated with metformin not only live longer but also retain better metabolic health, experiencing fewer instances of cancer, cardiovascular dysfunction, and cognitive impairment. Remarkably, these mice maintain their strength and mobility well into advanced age, vividly illustrating healthy aging.

Equally promising results have surfaced from studies on Caenorhabditis elegans (C. elegans), microscopic worms often used in aging research. In these tiny organisms, metformin prolongs lifespan by reshaping their gut microbiome and improving metabolic efficiency—highlighting an intriguing connection between microbial health and longevity, currently being explored in larger, more complex animals.

Among primates, metformin shows protective effects across multiple organ systems, including kidneys, lungs, skin, and brain. Especially noteworthy is its ability to reduce the buildup of senescent cells—often termed "zombie cells"—that persist in tissues, releasing harmful inflammatory compounds. By limiting these problematic cells, metformin may help preserve tissue health and delay systemic aging.

In humans, observational studies offer compelling insights. People with type 2 diabetes taking metformin often exhibit lower overall mortality rates than even non-diabetic individuals. This paradox has fueled intense scientific curiosity, suggesting metformin's benefits might extend broadly beyond glucose management. Some studies even propose that diabetics using metformin could live as long—or even longer—than healthy individuals who do not take the medication.

While fascinating, these findings remain correlative rather than conclusive. To definitively establish whether metformin actively slows human aging, rigorous interventional research—like the eagerly anticipated TAME Trial—is indispensable. Only through carefully designed clinical studies can we truly understand if metformin holds the key to a longer and healthier life for all.

The TAME Trial: A Defining Test for Metformin's Longevity Potential

Aging has long been viewed as an inevitable decline, yet emerging research raises the exciting possibility that it might be actively managed—or even slowed down. Investigating this transformative potential is the primary aim of the Targeting Aging with Metformin (TAME) Trial. Unlike traditional clinical trials that typically examine treatments for individual diseases, TAME is uniquely designed to test whether metformin can simultaneously delay the onset of multiple age-related conditions. If successful, this could fundamentally shift medical perspectives, repositioning aging from an unavoidable process into a modifiable risk factor and revolutionizing medicine's approach to age-related decline.

The potential implications of TAME extend beyond metformin. Should the trial provide convincing evidence that pharmacological interventions can slow aging, regulatory bodies like the FDA might officially recognize aging as a treatable condition. Such recognition could open a new chapter in medicine, paving the way not only for broader metformin use but also accelerating the development of innovative therapies explicitly aimed at prolonging years of good health, or "healthspan."

Nevertheless, conducting a trial like TAME poses significant challenges. Aging currently isn't classified as a disease, complicating regulatory approval for interventions explicitly targeting longevity. Moreover, human aging is inherently complex, influenced by a mosaic of genetic, environmental, and lifestyle factors, making it difficult to isolate and quantify metformin's precise impact. Unlike tightly controlled laboratory experiments, large-scale human studies require extensive follow-up periods, considerable funding, and diverse participant populations to yield definitive results.

If the TAME Trial proves successful despite these hurdles, the outcomes could be truly transformative. Demonstrating that an affordable, widely available medication can positively influence multiple aging pathways would significantly strengthen the argument for officially treating aging as a medical condition. Such a shift could catalyze the development of numerous advanced longevity therapies—from targeted interventions activating AMPK and inhibiting mTOR to specialized treatments designed to eliminate harmful senescent cells.

As research continues to advance, the TAME Trial represents a critical milestone, potentially reshaping how we understand and address aging. Regardless of whether metformin becomes a mainstay in longevity medicine or simply a pathway to more advanced interventions, the outcomes of TAME will unquestionably influence the future direction of aging research and medical innovation

Metformin and Exercise: Balancing Metabolic Benefits and Physical Adaptation

The relationship between metformin and exercise reveals a fascinating paradox. Each intervention individually enhances metabolic health, insulin sensitivity, and mitochondrial function; however, their combined effects don't always align predictably. Metformin, long known as a powerful metabolic regulator, interacts with many of the same cellular pathways activated by exercise, creating potential trade-offs. How these two powerful influences interact can differ widely between individuals, influenced by personal physiology, fitness goals, and metabolic health. Clearly understanding this intricate interplay is vital to effectively integrating metformin into an active lifestyle.

Exercise is among the most potent drivers of metabolic and muscular adaptations. It boosts insulin sensitivity, optimizes mitochondrial efficiency, and strengthens the body's response to oxidative stress—all crucial elements of long-term metabolic resilience. Yet, metformin also influences these pathways, sometimes complementing exercise-induced adaptations and sometimes hindering them. For some, metformin and exercise may harmonize beautifully, enhancing each other's beneficial effects, like instruments performing in perfect sync. For others, however, metformin may inadvertently blunt critical adaptations necessary for endurance, muscle growth, or energy efficiency—akin to a subtly discordant note disrupting an otherwise harmonious melody. Thoughtfully balancing these interactions helps ensure metformin supports, rather than interferes with, the benefits of regular physical activity.

Metformin's Influence on Exercise Adaptations

Metformin influences exercise adaptations through mechanisms that intersect with, yet distinctly differ from, those activated by physical activity. Picture metformin interacting with some of the same cellular "control panels" as exercise. For instance, metformin activates AMP-activated protein kinase (AMPK)—a sensor that boosts glucose uptake, fatty acid burning, and mitochondrial efficiency—enhancing metabolic health similarly to regular exercise. However, activating AMPK also inhibits the mechanistic Target of Rapamycin (mTOR), which is critical for muscle protein synthesis. Imagine pressing the accelerator while applying the brakes simultaneously; this dual action raises concerns, particularly for individuals aiming to increase muscle mass through resistance training.

Adding further complexity, metformin inhibits mitochondrial complex I, a vital enzyme responsible for ATP production—the energy source for muscles during exercise. Consider mitochondria as tiny power plants; metformin's interference could reduce energy availability during prolonged or intense endurance exercise. Casual exercisers may never notice this minor effect, but elite athletes or endurance-focused individuals might find it more noticeable.

Mixed Outcomes: When Metformin and Exercise Collide

The combined effects of metformin and exercise vary depending on factors such as exercise type, intensity, duration, and individual metabolic conditions. Some studies indicate that metformin may blunt the improvements in insulin sensitivity typically gained from exercise, highlighting that combining two beneficial interventions does not always produce additive advantages.

Regarding muscle growth, metformin's activation of AMPK and inhibition of mTOR could limit muscle mass and strength gains from resistance training. Research findings, however, remain inconsistent—some suggest reduced muscle growth, while others find minimal or no significant impact. This variability underscores the importance of personalized approaches, especially for older adults prioritizing functional strength and muscle preservation.

Who Benefits Most? Individual Considerations

Metformin's influence on exercise isn't uniform; it varies significantly based on age, metabolic health, and fitness goals. For older adults, maintaining strength and physical function is vital for quality of life and independence. If metformin interferes with muscle-building responses to exercise, it might be less suitable as a longevity intervention for those without metabolic concerns. Conversely, for those managing diabetes, prediabetes, or insulin resistance, metformin's ability to stabilize blood sugar and reduce inflammation might outweigh minor limitations on muscle adaptations. In these scenarios, combining metformin with moderate resistance training could effectively balance metabolic and muscular health.

Athletes and performance-focused individuals face different considerations. Metformin's effects on mTOR signaling and mitochondrial function might hinder muscular or endurance adaptations crucial for intensive or strength-focused training. Those committed to peak performance may strategically time metformin intake—such as taking it in the evening or on rest days—to minimize potential disruptions to training adaptations.

For most people exercising primarily for general health and longevity, these concerns become far less significant. Moderate activities, including walking, cycling, or modest resistance training, generally remain unaffected by metformin use. In these contexts, metformin provides substantial metabolic benefits, complementing rather than conflicting with a healthy, active lifestyle.

Metformin and Longevity: Final Reflections

Originally developed as a diabetes medication, metformin has emerged as one of the most intriguing candidates in longevity research. Its wide-ranging biological effects—including metabolic regulation, inflammation reduction, improved mitochondrial efficiency, and enhanced cellular maintenance—position it uniquely within aging science and preventive healthcare. More than a treatment for blood sugar management, metformin symbolizes a broader medical shift, reinforcing the idea that aging involves biological mechanisms potentially responsive to intervention.

Few medications match metformin's combination of affordability, established safety profile, and diverse physiological benefits, making it particularly attractive for longevity-focused studies. However, individual responses vary considerably based on factors such as metabolic health, genetics, lifestyle, and physical activity levels, emphasizing the necessity of personalized approaches. Those with insulin resistance or metabolic dysfunction may derive substantial benefits from metformin, whereas healthy adults aiming primarily for muscle growth or peak physical performance should carefully assess its trade-offs.

Current research efforts, including ongoing major clinical trials, will help determine metformin's ultimate role in influencing human aging. Even as scientists debate whether metformin will become central to longevity medicine or simply a foundation for more advanced therapeutic developments, its scientific and philosophical impact is undeniable. Moving forward, the key challenge lies not in choosing between pharmacological or lifestyle approaches but rather in thoughtfully integrating both strategies to comprehensively support a longer, healthier life.

CHAPTER 16

Boosting NAD+: NMN and NR in Cellular Rejuvenation

"Progress is not in enhancing what is, but in advancing toward what will be."
—KHALIL GIBRAN

NAD+ is an essential coenzyme deeply embedded in every cell of the body, playing a crucial role in maintaining life. As a powerful catalyst, NAD+ drives numerous biological processes necessary for cellular energy, vitality, and longevity. If cells lack sufficient NAD+, they begin to struggle—like engines deprived of fuel—disrupting energy production, DNA repair, and metabolic balance.

The Multifaceted Role of NAD+ in the Body

Envision NAD+ as your body's internal battery charger, continuously replenishing cellular energy reserves. Central to metabolism, NAD+ facilitates the production of ATP—the primary energy currency of cells—by transporting electrons through the mitochondrial electron transport chain. Just as a failing battery compromises the performance of electronic devices, reduced NAD+ levels can result in fatigue, sluggishness, and mental fog. Yet NAD+ serves more roles than just energy production. Your DNA functions like an invaluable manuscript, continuously exposed to environmental pollutants, metabolic waste, and daily cellular stressors. NAD+ activates specialized DNA-repair enzymes known as poly ADP-ribose polymerases (PARPs), diligent "editors" that carefully detect and correct DNA breaks. This essential editing preserves genetic integrity and protects against age-related mutations. When NAD+ levels fall, DNA repair slows, accelerating cellular aging.

Additionally, NAD+ partners closely with proteins called sirtuins—often described as guardians of cellular longevity. Sirtuins regulate stress responses, inflammation, and metabolism, but their activity hinges entirely upon NAD+. Elevated NAD+ levels significantly enhance sirtuin function, bolstering cellular resilience and slowing aging. Conversely, as NAD+ declines, sirtuin activity diminishes, intensifying oxidative stress and inflammation and ultimately impairing overall cellular function. NAD+ also plays a critical role in immune system regulation, particularly in managing chronic inflammation, known as "inflammaging." This low-grade, persistent inflammation silently damages tissues and contributes to conditions like cardiovascular disease, diabetes, and neurodegenerative disorders. Maintaining adequate NAD+ levels helps efficiently control inflammation, reducing systemic deterioration and mitigating age-related disease progression.

The NAD+ Decline: A Challenge of Aging

Despite its crucial roles, NAD+ naturally declines as we age. By middle age, NAD+ concentrations may decrease by nearly half, manifesting as persistent fatigue, slower recovery times after exertion, and diminished physical performance. As NAD+ reserves decline, critical cellular repair mechanisms become compromised, allowing genetic damage to accumulate more quickly, accelerating aging and increasing vulnerability to chronic diseases. Reduced NAD+ further weakens sirtuin activation, exacerbating oxidative stress and chronic inflammation—conditions closely associated with heart disease, diabetes, and neurodegenerative illnesses. In response, researchers are actively pursuing innovative strategies to restore NAD+ levels, from dietary supplements and lifestyle changes to advanced therapeutic approaches. These strategies aim to replenish this essential cellular resource, enhancing innate physiological resilience and potentially transforming age-related challenges into opportunities for improved health and vitality.

NAD+ Boosters: NMN and NR–Unlocking Cellular Vitality

Recognizing the importance of replenishing declining NAD+, scientists have focused extensively on two key compounds: Nicotinamide Mononucleotide (NMN) and Nicotinamide Riboside (NR). Direct NAD+ supplementation often fails due to poor absorption; however, NMN and NR efficiently boost NAD+ levels by acting as essential building blocks. NMN swiftly converts into NAD+, providing an efficient pathway for cellular rejuvenation. While naturally found in foods like broccoli, edamame, and avocado, the dietary amounts are too low for meaningful NAD+ elevation. Supplemental NMN particularly benefits high-energy-demanding tissues such as muscle, liver, and the cardiovascular system. In contrast, NR requires an additional metabolic conversion, first transforming into NMN before becoming NAD+. Found naturally in trace quantities in milk and yeast, NR efficiently elevates NAD+ levels, especially in neural and metabolic tissues. Its ability to cross the blood-brain barrier uniquely positions it as beneficial for cognitive health, memory, and clarity during aging.

Both NMN and NR support mitochondrial function, improving glucose metabolism and insulin sensitivity, potentially reducing risks related to insulin resistance and type 2 diabetes. NMN notably promotes cardiovascular endurance and vascular health, while NR demonstrates distinct advantages for neuroprotection and cognitive function. Typical daily dosages for NMN and NR range from 250 mg to 500 mg and are generally well-tolerated, though higher doses may cause mild digestive discomfort. Animal studies suggest possible lifespan extension, yet definitive conclusions require further human research. Lifestyle choices also significantly impact NAD+ levels. Regular exercise, intermittent fasting, and caloric restriction stimulate NAD+ biosynthesis and mitochondrial efficiency. In contrast, alcohol consumption rapidly reduces NAD+, underscoring the importance of mindful lifestyle decisions to maintain cellular health. By thoughtfully combining targeted supplementation with intentional lifestyle practices, we can effectively support NAD+ levels, promoting lasting cellular health and sustained vitality throughout life.

Sustaining Cellular Vitality with NAD+

The evolving science of NAD+ underscores practical strategies for cellular wellness. While the foundational science is sound, definitive evidence for extending human lifespan or dramatically reversing aging is still under investigation. Nonetheless, proactive replenishment of NAD+, through carefully selected supplements such as NMN and NR, offers tangible benefits supported by current research. However, as will be emphasized throughout this book, lasting cellular vitality depends fundamentally on foundational habits—regular physical activity, restorative sleep, and a nutrient-rich diet.

Integrating these lifestyle elements with targeted supplementation provides a comprehensive approach, optimizing cellular resilience and enhancing overall well-being. As our understanding of NAD+ continues to expand, sustaining robust cellular function becomes not just aspirational but realistically achievable, empowering us to maintain physiological resilience throughout life.

CHAPTER 17

Cellular Rejuvenation: Senolytics, Acarbose, and Telomerase in Aging Science

"For age is opportunity no less than youth itself, though in another dress, and as the evening twilight fades away, the sky is filled with stars, invisible by day."
—Henry Wadsworth Longfellow

As the science of aging advances, researchers are increasingly turning their attention to an emerging strategy: the targeted removal of senescent cells. These so-called "zombie cells" have lost their ability to divide, yet they stubbornly linger in tissues, disrupting function, fueling inflammation, and accelerating biological decline. While senescence plays a protective role in early life, preventing the unchecked growth of damaged cells, its accumulation over time becomes a detrimental force. Instead of supporting tissue integrity, senescent cells secrete inflammatory molecules, hinder regeneration, and contribute to organ deterioration.

To counteract this process, scientists have developed senolytics, a class of compounds designed to eliminate senescent cells and restore cellular balance. By removing these dysfunctional cells, senolytics aim to reduce inflammation, enhance tissue repair, and potentially extend both healthspan and lifespan. Yet cellular rejuvenation is not solely about eliminating the old—it also requires preserving and optimizing the function of healthy cells. This chapter explores how senolytics work, the expanding array of compounds targeting cellular senescence, and complementary strategies such as telomerase activation and metabolic regulation, which together provide a multi-pronged approach to longevity.

The Dual Nature of Cellular Senescence

Cellular senescence is a double-edged sword—a safeguard against cancer and uncontrolled cell division, yet over time, a key driver of chronic disease and aging. When cells experience irreparable damage due to oxidative stress, DNA mutations, or repeated replication, they enter a senescent state, halting division to prevent the spread of potentially harmful errors. Ideally, these cells undergo apoptosis, a self-destruct mechanism that removes them from the body. However, many evade this fate, persisting within tissues where they interfere with normal cellular processes and create an inflammatory microenvironment.

A primary culprit in this dysfunction is the senescence-associated secretory phenotype (SASP)—a toxic cocktail of inflammatory cytokines, proteases, and growth factors. Rather than lying dormant, senescent cells actively alter their surroundings, driving chronic inflammation, tissue breakdown, and immune system dysfunction. This ongoing inflammatory state—often called "inflammaging"—is directly implicated in cardiovascular disease, arthritis, neurodegeneration, and metabolic disorders.

Adding to the problem, senescent cells do not operate in isolation. They send distress signals that can induce neighboring healthy cells to enter senescence prematurely, creating a chain reaction of cellular dysfunction. Compounding matters further, the immune system's ability to clear senescent cells declines with age, allowing them to accumulate and exert an ever-greater burden on tissues.

Senolytics: Clearing the Path for Regeneration

Senolytics approach aging in a unique way by selectively targeting and eliminating senescent cells, enabling the body to reclaim tissue function and restore cellular homeostasis. These compounds trigger apoptosis, reawakening the natural self-destruct process that senescent cells have skillfully evaded. Their removal frees up biological space, allowing younger, more functional cells to flourish.

Beyond cellular housekeeping, the system-wide effects of senolytics are substantial. By reducing SASP-driven inflammation, these compounds may lower the risk of chronic diseases, enhance immune resilience, and support healthier organ function. Preclinical studies have already demonstrated significant improvements in tissue regeneration, reduced markers of systemic inflammation, and even evidence of age-related reversal in some biological functions.

Not all senescent cells are detrimental. Some play essential roles in wound healing, tissue remodeling, and even preventing fibrosis. Completely eradicating them without discretion could impair the body's natural repair mechanisms. For this reason, researchers are exploring intermittent dosing strategies, where senolytics are administered in carefully timed cycles, maximizing benefits while avoiding unintended consequences.

Innovating Cellular Health: The Next Generation of Senolytics

The field of senolytics is expanding rapidly, uncovering a diverse array of pharmaceutical and naturally derived compounds beyond the well-established Dasatinib, Quercetin, and Fisetin. These emerging candidates operate through distinct mechanisms, reflecting the complexity of cellular senescence and the potential for multifaceted therapeutic interventions.

Among the leading pharmaceutical senolytics is Navitoclax (ABT-263), initially developed as an anti-cancer agent. It inhibits BCL-2 proteins, disrupting survival pathways that allow senescent cells to persist. While promising in early studies, its toxicity to platelets and other blood cells remains a significant challenge.

One of the most promising experimental senolytics currently under investigation is FOXO4-DRI. This peptide is carefully designed to disrupt the interaction between FOXO4 and p53 proteins, thereby reactivating apoptosis in senescent cells. Animal studies have shown compelling results. Researchers observed significant improvements in organ functionality, enhanced tissue resilience, and even visibly rejuvenated physical appearance. While these findings offer intriguing glimpses into future possibilities, caution remains essential. Definitive evidence of safety and efficacy awaits results from extensive human trials.

Natural compounds also provide intriguing alternatives. Apigenin, a flavonoid found abundantly in parsley, chamomile, and celery, exhibits potential senolytic activity. Alongside this property, it offers notable anti-inflammatory and antioxidant benefits. Similarly promising is EGCG (Epigallocatechin Gallate) from green tea. This compound demonstrates modest senolytic effects in addition to its well-known anti-inflammatory and cardioprotective roles. Although these natural substances appear encouraging, current evidence primarily arises from laboratory and animal studies. Human studies are needed to confirm their true therapeutic potential.

Collectively, these developments illuminate exciting new paths in our quest to address aging at a cellular level. These compounds could significantly expand the therapeutic toolkit. They offer hope for preserving cellular health and possibly extending our years of wellness. Nevertheless, their promise is balanced by the necessity of rigorous validation. Only through careful evaluation can these fascinating discoveries move from intriguing possibilities to trusted, practical solutions.

Exploring the Synergy: Senolytics and Telomerase Activation in Aging Research

While senolytics work to remove damaged cells, telomerase activators focus on preserving and extending the lifespan of healthy ones. These two approaches represent distinct strategies targeting the aging process from opposite ends. Senolytics clear senescent cells, which contribute to inflammation and degeneration, while telomerase activation aims to sustain cellular vitality by rebuilding telomeres—the protective caps at the ends of chromosomes. Telomeres naturally shorten with each cell division, and as they diminish, they ultimately lead to cellular aging and dysfunction. Telomerase, however, counteracts this decline by rebuilding these telomeres, thus prolonging cellular lifespan and bolstering the body's capacity to maintain healthy tissues over time.

Telomerase activation is particularly promising for high-turnover tissues such as the immune system, skin, and gut lining, which rely on continuous cell division to stay functional. By supporting this process, telomerase activation can delay aging and enhance the regenerative capacity of these tissues, offering significant potential for extending the health of critical systems.

Yet, telomerase activation is not without its risks. While the extension of telomeres can improve cellular longevity, excessive activation comes with a notable cancer risk. Tumors often exploit telomerase to enable uncontrolled cell growth, and overactivation could inadvertently promote tumorigenesis. Future therapies must find a way to balance telomere maintenance, activating telomerase in a manner that supports healthy cell function without triggering malignancy.

Combining senolytics with telomerase activation could offer a powerful dual strategy to combat aging. By targeting damaged cells and simultaneously preserving the health of healthy ones, these therapies may hold the key to slowing aging and extending healthspan. Together, they provide a pathway not just for living longer, but for living with greater health—avoiding the frailty and decline that often accompany the aging process.

Acarbose: A Multi-Pathway Approach to Longevity

Beyond the realm of cellular renewal, metabolic regulation plays a pivotal role in healthy aging. One particularly intriguing intervention is acarbose—a drug originally developed to manage type 2 diabetes—now drawing attention for its potential to enhance lifespan and optimize metabolic function.

Acarbose works by slowing the digestion of carbohydrates in the small intestine, where it inhibits alpha-glucosidase, an enzyme responsible for breaking down starches and sugars. By doing so, it prevents sharp post-meal glucose spikes, easing the metabolic burden placed on the body after eating. This effect helps protect against oxidative stress, a contributor to cellular aging, and reduces the formation of advanced glycation end-products (AGEs)—harmful compounds that form when sugars bind to proteins, accelerating tissue aging and the deterioration of metabolic processes.

But acarbose's influence doesn't end there. It also impacts the gut microbiome, that vast ecosystem of bacteria living in our intestines. As acarbose ferments in the large intestine, it creates a favorable environment for beneficial bacteria, increasing the production of short-chain fatty acids (SCFAs) like butyrate. These SCFAs play a crucial role in boosting insulin sensitivity, reducing chronic inflammation, and improving overall gut health. In turn, they contribute to metabolic stability and help counteract age-related decline. Studies in animal models have linked these effects to longer lifespans and greater vitality, showcasing the far-reaching benefits of this compound.

Targeting Aging through Integrated Cellular Strategies

The convergence of senolytics, telomerase activators, and metabolic regulators is reframing how we approach aging at the cellular level. These interventions target key aspects of aging through complementary mechanisms: senolytics clear dysfunctional senescent cells that fuel chronic inflammation and tissue degeneration; telomerase activators work to maintain telomere length, supporting the regenerative capacity of cells; and metabolic regulators optimize critical processes like glucose metabolism and insulin sensitivity, both of which are integral to cellular health.

Together, these therapies form a promising strategy for enhancing the duration of healthy, active life by addressing the underlying causes of age-related decline. Although research is still in its early stages, particularly in human trials, the potential to slow aging and mitigate age-related diseases is becoming increasingly clear.

CHAPTER 18

Non-Pharmacological Biohacks: Effective Optimization Without Medication

"The only way to discover the limits of the possible is to venture a little way past them into the impossible."
—ARTHUR C. CLARKE

Aging should no longer be regarded as an inevitable, steady decline—like sand slipping through an hourglass. Instead, scientists increasingly recognize it as a dynamic, adaptable process that we can actively shape through intentional, strategic interventions. While pharmaceuticals and nutritional supplements have traditionally dominated the pursuit of longevity, an intriguing new frontier is capturing attention: biohacking. Biohacking promises to awaken the body's innate regenerative abilities by harnessing environmental and sensory influences rather than relying exclusively on chemical solutions. Non-pharmacological biohacking applies sophisticated technologies and therapeutic techniques to fine-tune cellular functions, strengthen biological resilience, and elevate overall wellness. These innovative interventions often complement traditional medicine or open entirely new pathways toward improved health and longevity.

As biohacking continues to evolve, it shifts our perspective on aging, challenging traditional views and opening new possibilities. Unlike pharmaceuticals—which target precise molecular pathways like arrows hitting defined targets—non-pharmacological biohacks broadly engage fundamental biological systems through carefully curated environmental and physical inputs. When skillfully applied, these powerful yet natural triggers stimulate cellular repair, optimize energy metabolism, and sharpen cognitive and physical performance, all without the systemic side effects common with pharmaceuticals.

However, the effectiveness of these methods can vary widely. Some approaches are backed by robust scientific evidence and already enjoy widespread use, while others remain experimental, awaiting further scientific validation. As ongoing research progresses, eager early adopters are integrating these approaches into their daily lives, hoping to tap into their promising potential to sustain health and vitality. Yet responsible implementation calls for a thoughtful, evidence-based approach, blending enthusiasm and curiosity with critical thinking. Each person's individual responses and specific health needs must guide judicious application.

Perhaps the most inviting aspect of non-pharmacologic biohacking is its ease of access. Many of these interventions can seamlessly weave into daily routines, providing practical, low-risk avenues toward better health and longer life. Simple lifestyle adjustments—such as optimizing natural daily rhythms or gradually introducing environmental stimuli—can yield clear, tangible benefits, sidestepping the complexities or potential risks often associated with pharmaceuticals.

Non-pharmacological biohacking is rapidly emerging as a core component of contemporary longevity strategies, evolving in tandem with increasingly sophisticated and experimentally driven pharmacologic therapies. Although many of these cutting-edge interventions remain under investigation, their development signals a meaningful shift in how we understand and influence the biology of aging. These breakthroughs seek not only to extend life but to transform its quality—expanding the scope of human health in ways that were, until recently, beyond scientific reach.

The future holds exciting promise as biohacking, science, and technology continue to converge seamlessly. Anchored firmly in scientific principles and strategically combined with proven lifestyle practices, these emerging capabilities can unlock humanity's potential to continuously extend both healthspan and lifespan.

Enhancing Longevity Through Real-Time Health Tracking

Imagine navigating a cross-country journey guided only by occasional road signs. This scenario mirrors traditional health management, characterized by sporadic doctor visits and annual physical exams. Today, advanced health tracking technologies offer continuous monitoring of vital indicators such as glucose levels, heart rate variability, sleep quality, stress, hormone fluctuations, and metabolic function. These real-time insights empower proactive, informed decision-making rather than reactive interventions.

Wearable devices—smartwatches, fitness trackers, biometric rings—deliver ongoing feedback about heart rate variability, sleep patterns, oxygen saturation, and physical activity. Such immediate data directly influence daily lifestyle choices around fitness, rest, and recovery. Yet, wearable accuracy varies with sensor placement, skin type, movement, and individual physiology. Periodic clinical evaluations and laboratory tests can complement wearable data, forming a robust and comprehensive health profile.

Continuous glucose monitors (CGMs), small sensors placed beneath the skin, provide a detailed picture of metabolic responses. Users can vividly observe how dietary choices, exercise routines, stress, and sleep impact blood glucose levels. Maintaining stable glucose levels not only helps prevent metabolic disorders like diabetes but also sustains energy, mental clarity, and overall well-being. CGM data supports precise dietary and behavioral adjustments for long-term metabolic health.

Metabolic tracking technologies, including respiratory analysis tools, measure indicators like resting metabolic rate and respiratory exchange ratio (RER). These metrics show precisely whether fats or carbohydrates predominantly fuel one's daily activities, creating an individualized nutritional and exercise blueprint. Athletes and those seeking optimal energy levels and metabolic flexibility find this particularly valuable.

Hormone assessments, conducted through saliva, blood, or urine tests, can detect nuanced shifts that influence mood, energy levels, metabolism, cognitive function, and overall well-being. Declines in hormones associated with aging—such as testosterone and estrogen—often lead to fatigue, fluctuations in weight, and cognitive difficulties. Regular hormonal monitoring allows for timely lifestyle adjustments, targeted supplementation, or medical interventions, helping to maintain hormonal balance and preserve optimal function.

Advanced sleep technologies like EEG headbands, smart mattresses, and specialized sleep trackers precisely analyze sleep stages, movements, and heart rate variability. These devices pinpoint factors disrupting restful sleep, empowering users to make targeted improvements—optimizing bedroom conditions, refining bedtime routines, or managing stress more effectively. Enhanced sleep quality supports cognitive performance, hormonal balance, immune health, and longevity, transforming sleep into an active cornerstone of sustained wellness.

The real value of real-time health tracking emerges when you thoughtfully apply insights from continuous monitoring, converting everyday data into practical habits that support lasting health and improved longevity.

Integrating and Transforming Health Data with Professional Guidance

Personalized medicine redefines health—not as isolated, disconnected data points, but as a cohesive narrative derived from diverse streams of information. Real-time tracking technologies continuously highlight critical indicators such as glucose levels, heart rate variability, sleep patterns, hormonal fluctuations, and metabolic function. Shifting from periodic snapshots to ongoing insights, this approach crafts an evolving, precise portrait of individual well-being, empowering informed and timely decisions.

However, abundant data alone does not automatically lead to better health outcomes. Without skilled interpretation and appropriate context, continuous streams of metrics can quickly overwhelm or mislead. For example, reacting impulsively to a short-term glucose spike or a single restless night of sleep might obscure deeper, more significant health patterns.

This challenge highlights the essential role of professional guidance. Healthcare providers serve as interpreters, translating complex data into clear, actionable strategies. Their expertise enables them to distinguish fleeting anomalies from meaningful, persistent patterns that genuinely require intervention. An occasional disrupted night's sleep likely demands no immediate adjustments, whereas chronic sleep disturbances signal a clear need for careful attention.

When expertly interpreted and strategically integrated with professional insights, real-time data becomes a powerful resource. This intentional fusion guides deliberate, informed actions rather than impulsive reactions, supporting sustainable and personalized improvements in health and longevity. Ultimately, this balanced partnership between data and skilled guidance ensures continuous information effectively translates into lasting, meaningful enhancements to overall well-being.

AI-Driven Health Platforms: Revolutionizing Personalized Wellness

Artificial intelligence is disrupting traditional health care through its extraordinary capacity to analyze vast amounts of health data. Like a seasoned investigator, AI examines streams of information from wearables, biomarkers, and genetic testing, identifying intricate connections that previously went unnoticed. These sophisticated, AI-driven platforms move beyond conventional analysis, revealing complex patterns and relationships hidden within immense datasets. Personalized recommendations emerge—targeted nutrition plans, optimized exercise routines, effective recovery strategies, and precise metabolic adjustments—unlocking health possibilities that once seemed unattainable.

Yet, harnessing the immense potential of AI in health optimization comes with critical challenges. The quality of AI-driven recommendations depends on accurate data inputs, ongoing algorithm refinement, and thorough validation processes. Privacy concerns loom large, as biometric and genetic information raises important questions regarding secure and ethical use. Ensuring equitable access to these powerful AI-driven tools is crucial. Furthermore, addressing algorithmic biases is essential. Maintaining transparency in AI applications is another vital step toward fostering trust and accountability.

As AI continues to advance, its impact reaches far beyond biohacking. From predictive analytics and early disease detection to precision medicine and proactive health management, AI is positioned to usher in a new era in longevity science. A more extensive exploration of AI's expanding role in shaping the future of health and aging is covered in a dedicated chapter of this book.

Real-Time Stress and Cognitive Function Monitoring

Stress is like waves in the ocean: gentle ones are manageable and even calming, yet left unchecked, they can grow powerful and overwhelming. Understanding the intricate relationship between stress and cognitive performance is essential for maintaining mental clarity and emotional balance. Wearable neurofeedback devices and real-time stress trackers provide continuous snapshots of key physiological indicators—such as heart rate variability, brainwave activity, and cortisol fluctuations. With these insights, it's possible to swiftly identify stress triggers, cognitive dips, and lifestyle patterns that influence productivity, decision-making, and overall mental sharpness.

Recognizing your unique stress patterns opens the door to targeted interventions that sharpen focus, enhance mental agility, and stabilize emotions. Techniques such as guided breathing exercises, structured meditation, or intentional lifestyle adjustments help regulate your body's stress responses, alleviating chronic strain on your nervous system. Embracing real-time monitoring transforms mental wellness from reactive to proactive, fostering enduring cognitive resilience and emotional adaptability.

Psychological and Behavioral Biohacking: Enhancing Mental Resilience Through Technology

Imagine your mind as an intricate ecosystem—a dynamic landscape thriving on careful attention and mindful cultivation. Biohacking, once primarily concerned with physical health, has expanded significantly to encompass mental and emotional well-being. Today, advanced technologies and scientifically validated methods empower us to fortify cognitive abilities, boost emotional resilience, and enhance psychological health.

Neurofeedback technology, employing electroencephalogram (EEG) devices, opens a window directly into the intricate rhythms of the brain. By visualizing brainwave patterns in real-time, you can consciously refine neural responses, sharpening focus, easing anxiety, and boosting cognitive adaptability. With consistent practice, these beneficial mental states become more natural, improving mental clarity, sleep quality, memory, and resilience against stress-induced cognitive decline.

Further pushing cognitive boundaries, transcranial electrical stimulation (tES) and transcranial magnetic stimulation (TMS) offer innovative possibilities. These non-invasive brain stimulation techniques modulate neural activity through precise electrical or magnetic pulses. tES is designed for safe at-home use, enhancing neuroplasticity and learning capacity, while TMS, typically provided in clinical settings, effectively addresses severe cognitive and mood disorders, including depression. As ongoing research and clinical validation progress, these methods emerge as potent strategies for maintaining cognitive health and emotional well-being.

Artificial intelligence has advanced cognitive enhancement through digital therapeutics and tailored apps. Far from routine mental drills, these interactive, dynamic programs adjust their challenges in response to your performance, much like a personal trainer adapting workouts. These targeted exercises enhance memory, sharpen problem-solving abilities, and accelerate processing speed, proactively sustaining mental agility and reducing the risk of cognitive decline.

Biofeedback bridges the gap between conscious thought and underlying physiological processes. Real-time visualization of bodily functions—such as heart rate, muscle tension, and breathing—enables active control over stress responses. When integrated with mindfulness practices or guided breathing exercises, biofeedback fosters mental resilience, emotional balance, and psychological stability.

Immersive technologies, such as virtual reality (VR) and augmented reality (AR), offer vivid cognitive enrichment experiences. By creating engaging, interactive environments, these tools stimulate spatial awareness, enhance concentration, and sharpen problem-solving capabilities. VR is particularly valuable for exposure therapy, providing safe settings to confront and manage fears or anxieties, effectively reducing emotional reactivity and enhancing adaptability.

Integrating these psychological biohacking technologies into daily life resembles skillfully adjusting sails to navigate life's shifting currents. Embracing these innovations alongside evidence-based practices may foster sustained mental resilience, emotional wellness, and enduring cognitive vitality.

Personalized Nutrition and Gut Microbiome Analysis

Within each of us lies a microscopic world, vibrant and complex as a flourishing garden. It's teeming with diverse organisms, each vital to sustaining the entire ecosystem. Recent advances in gut microbiome testing have shed new light on this intricate environment. These developments offer unprecedented insights into how deeply the microbiome influences health and longevity. Through microbiome sequencing, scientists now clearly see how specific bacterial compositions and activities impact digestion, metabolism, and immune function. These beneficial microorganisms aid nutrient absorption, regulate energy levels, and produce short-chain fatty acids (SCFAs). SCFAs are essential molecules, critical for efficient metabolism and effective inflammation management. Certain helpful bacteria even demonstrate the potential to improve blood sugar control, enhance digestion, and support weight management. Conversely, microbial imbalances have been associated with insulin resistance, obesity, and other metabolic disorders.

Moreover, the gut microbiome's influence extends far beyond metabolism alone. It serves as a central regulator of the immune system, maintains inflammatory balance, and even influences mental well-being through the intriguing gut-brain axis. Reduced microbial diversity has been linked to increased inflammation, mood disorders, and cognitive decline—underscoring the importance of nurturing a diverse and resilient microbiome to support healthy aging.

Microbiome sequencing is a powerful biohacking tool, providing precise measurements and clear insights into gut health. By interpreting personalized microbiome profiles, you can strategically adjust diet and lifestyle to cultivate microbial balance. This proactive, data-driven approach enhances metabolic function, strengthens immunity, and promotes overall wellness. Ultimately, microbiome analysis becomes more than information—it transforms into an actionable strategy for longevity.

Although microbiome science holds considerable promise for enhancing longevity, it remains an evolving field that requires careful interpretation of test results. Personalized dietary recommendations derived from microbiome profiles offer significant potential; however, they should be thoughtfully integrated into comprehensive health strategies that include genetic, lifestyle, and environmental considerations. Healthcare professionals, acting as skilled gardeners, can expertly interpret microbiome data and guide personalized interventions to optimize metabolic function, strengthen immunity, and support sustained well-being throughout the aging process.

Genetic and Epigenetic Testing: Unlocking Personalized Longevity Strategies

Your genetic blueprint serves as an inherited map, outlining possible paths your health might follow. Genetic testing can reveal predispositions to age-related conditions such as cardiovascular disease, diabetes, neurodegeneration, and cancer. Identifying specific markers—like APOE ε4, associated with Alzheimer's disease, or MTHFR, influencing methylation and folate metabolism—provides powerful insights. Equipped with this knowledge, people can adopt targeted lifestyle strategies, dietary modifications, tailored supplementation, and proactive medical screenings. Nevertheless, genetic predispositions represent probabilities, not certainties; lifestyle and environmental factors significantly influence health outcomes.

Epigenetic testing enriches this genetic foundation, demonstrating how external factors—diet, exercise, stress, and environmental exposures—actively influence gene expression. Epigenetic mechanisms, including DNA methylation and histone modifications, act as biological switches adjusting gene activity without changing the DNA sequence. Epigenetic markers offer insights into biological age, frequently differing from chronological age and more accurately reflecting cellular health. Although promising, epigenetic assessments remain developmental, with interpretations varying widely among laboratories and evolving clinical consensus.

Integrating genetic and epigenetic insights creates a comprehensive, personalized longevity strategy. For instance, someone genetically predisposed to cardiovascular disease can proactively adopt heart-healthy dietary habits and customized exercise routines. Regular epigenetic testing then provides actionable feedback, allowing timely adjustments to optimize long-term wellness.

While genetic testing captures inherited traits, epigenetic assessments offer dynamic, actionable insights. Careful interpretation, guided by collaboration with healthcare providers or genetic counselors, ensures interventions remain evidence-based and personalized. Ultimately, integrating genetic and epigenetic testing empowers informed decision-making, fostering improved wellness, reduced risk of chronic disease, and deeper understanding of one's unique aging journey.

Genetics and epigenetics, foundational yet rapidly evolving fields, warrant deeper exploration. In an upcoming chapter, we delve further into their intricate roles, examining groundbreaking research and emerging technologies to unlock even greater potential for molecular precision in longevity planning.

Environmental Biohacks: Harnessing Natural Forces

Our bodies naturally synchronize with environmental rhythms, shaping metabolism, mood, sleep, and overall health. Environmental biohacking taps into these innate connections, ranging from scientifically supported techniques to exploratory practices awaiting deeper validation.

Consider deuterium-depleted water (DDW), a specialized form of water refined to contain reduced levels of the heavy hydrogen isotope deuterium. Early evidence hints that lower deuterium concentrations might boost mitochondrial efficiency, enhancing cellular energy production and reducing oxidative stress—both critical factors in aging and chronic disease. While intriguing, DDW remains expensive and requires further robust clinical studies before widespread adoption.

Circadian lighting systems offer a practical yet elegant solution to synchronize internal biological clocks with external daylight cycles. Bright, blue-enriched morning light gradually awakens the mind, enhancing alertness and cognition, while softer, amber-hued evening light promotes relaxation and melatonin production, preparing the body for restful sleep. These systems are particularly beneficial for shift workers or people living in regions with significant fluctuations in natural daylight.

Imagine the refreshing sense of clarity felt near waterfalls or dense forests; these environments are rich in negative ions—charged particles associated with mood enhancement, cognitive clarity, and respiratory wellness. Research suggests negative ions may alleviate depression symptoms, boost oxygen uptake, and enhance indoor air quality, though these claims await further rigorous studies.

Grounding, or earthing, provides another accessible approach—simply walking barefoot outdoors reconnects us directly with the Earth's electrical energy. Advocates report reduced inflammation, balanced cortisol levels, and improved sleep quality from this direct earth-body contact. Though ongoing research continues, grounding's intuitive simplicity and low cost make it an appealing practice for enhancing well-being.

Electromagnetic field (EMF) shielding addresses growing concerns about radiation from ubiquitous digital devices like smartphones and Wi-Fi routers. While regulatory authorities affirm typical exposure levels as safe, precautionary measures such as specialized shielding fabrics or device distancing remain popular. Preliminary studies and anecdotal experiences suggest benefits like improved sleep quality and decreased fatigue, though definitive scientific conclusions are still awaited. Practical strategies, such as reducing device proximity during sleep, offer sensible, balanced approaches.

Intentionally integrating environmental biohacks alongside foundational health practices—nutrition, exercise, and sleep hygiene—creates a comprehensive strategy for enhancing vitality. Approached with balanced curiosity and grounded in scientific evidence, these practices align internal rhythms with external environments, fostering resilience, vitality, and sustained wellness.

Ethical and Privacy Considerations in Health Data Collection

Health-tracking technologies are swiftly reshaping our understanding of wellness, much like explorers charting new, promising territories. Wearable devices, biomarker testing, and genetic profiling generate vast troves of personalized health data, providing unprecedented insights into longevity and overall health. However, with innovation comes significant ethical responsibility—particularly concerning data security, informed consent, and responsible use.

Transparency is essential. People must clearly understand how their personal health data is gathered, shared, and applied, empowering them to confidently engage with these advancements without compromising privacy. Digital health platforms integrate diverse data streams into detailed profiles, enabling highly personalized longevity strategies. Yet extensive data collection also introduces risks—potential breaches, unauthorized access, or misuse by third parties like insurers or employers.

Robust protections, including advanced encryption, anonymization methods, and strict regulations on commercial usage, help secure sensitive information. Without these measures, trust could erode, undermining the potential for proactive health management.

Nonetheless, personalized health data offers considerable benefits. Advanced analytics and artificial intelligence facilitate early disease detection, precision treatments, and proactive aging management. Real-time tracking provides immediate, actionable insights, allowing precise adjustments to daily health choices. Achieving these benefits requires careful balance—leveraging powerful data insights while diligently upholding ethical standards and privacy.

As health-tracking technologies evolve, ethical and privacy guidelines must progress simultaneously. Thoughtful oversight and responsible data management support informed health decisions, ensuring innovations enhance quality of life without sacrificing personal autonomy.

A Vision for the Future

Biohacking isn't a quest for immortality or an eternal fountain of youth. Instead, it embodies a thoughtful, lifelong journey of self-discovery and continual improvement, deeply rooted in scientific progress and personal responsibility. Successful biohackers appreciate that genuine advancement arises from disciplined and flexible practices, respecting the profound complexities inherent in human biology. True achievement emerges from a balanced approach—embracing innovation yet steadfastly adhering to reliable, evidence-based health principles.

As longevity science increasingly merges with technological advancements, the ability to influence aging becomes more attainable each year. While dramatic life extension or outright reversal of aging remains distant, biohacking currently provides effective methods for optimizing health, enhancing adaptability, and improving overall well-being. Nevertheless, approaching biohacking methods demands significant caution and informed skepticism. Certain practices, despite holding intriguing promise, remain experimental and lack extensive scientific validation. Emphasizing cautious exploration does not deter curiosity; instead, it encourages mindful inquiry, wise decision-making, and attentive monitoring of individual experiences.

Moreover, the potential of biohacking extends well beyond individual benefits. As more people proactively embrace strategies for healthy aging, broader social attitudes are likely to evolve. Longstanding perceptions of aging as a period marked by decline and limitation could shift toward recognizing lifelong opportunities for renewal, continuous growth, and personal development. Such a shift would influence healthcare priorities, workplace practices, and societal views about aging itself. Ultimately, this evolving perspective frames aging not as an obstacle, but as a meaningful and dynamic phase filled with possibility.

Part IV
Next-Generation Longevity— Personalized Health and Revolutionary Innovation

"The best way to predict the future is to create it."
—Peter Drucker

Longevity is no longer something to passively accept; it has become an active pursuit, shaped by the interplay of biology, lifestyle choices, and scientific advancements. Recent breakthroughs—including personalized diagnostics, precision medicine, and innovative therapeutic approaches—are transforming not only how we prevent disease and maintain health but also extending human lifespan in ways scarcely imaginable just a few decades ago.

Envision a future where illness is identified and addressed before it can fully manifest—where nanotechnology repairs cellular damage at its origin, and therapies are tailored precisely to each person's genetic blueprint. The outdated notion of aging as an unavoidable decline is rapidly yielding to a more dynamic perspective. Although biological aging remains intrinsic, the pace of decline no longer follows a fixed trajectory. Scientific developments increasingly enable us to slow, alter, and in some cases even reverse aspects of senescence. Once speculative, these advances are becoming tangible realities as pioneering methods challenge conventional boundaries and alter our perceptions of aging.

These extraordinary developments carry significant responsibilities. As transformative solutions become integrated into everyday life, careful consideration of their ethical and societal implications is crucial. The expanding role of personalized health tracking and AI-driven diagnostics requires deliberate attention to data privacy, equitable access, and the long-term consequences for safety and personal autonomy. Ultimately, progress will be measured not by the length of our lives, but by the richness of experiences, quality of relationships, and sense of fulfillment defining those additional years.

In this section, we explore groundbreaking innovations revolutionizing longevity science. From genetic reprogramming and advanced diagnostics to cellular rejuvenation, these advancements push the frontiers of possibility. We'll examine how such developments not only prolong life but radically alter our understanding and approach to aging.

These achievements represent only part of the equation. Their true potential lies not merely in adopting novel approaches but in effectively integrating them into daily routines. This leads us into the final two chapters, essential for translating breakthroughs from theory into practice. By building your Longevity Team and crafting a personalized Longevity Plan, you'll take decisive steps toward making these cutting-edge strategies practical, sustainable, and impactful.

The pursuit of longevity reflects a desire not simply to extend existence, but to cultivate a life worthy of its length. It is a journey driven by curiosity, exploration, and the aspiration to exceed perceived limits. As research accelerates and new discoveries emerge, we stand at the dawn of a new era in human health—one in which aging is no longer dictated solely by time, but shaped by our collective determination to transform the future.

CHAPTER 19

Regenerative Medicine: Unlocking Your Body's Healing Potential

"What lies behind us and what lies before us are tiny matters compared to what lies within us."
—RALPH WALDO EMERSON

Medicine today is experiencing an inspiring transformation—from managing symptoms and slowing decline to actively encouraging healing and renewal. At the forefront of this remarkable shift is regenerative medicine, a field dedicated to tapping into the body's natural power to repair itself and even reverse certain aspects of aging. This approach offers significant possibilities for extending human longevity and enhancing our quality of life.

However, this compelling vision is accompanied by complexities. Regenerative medicine is an evolving frontier, filled with uncertainties about long-term outcomes, ethical considerations, shifting regulatory landscapes, and limited accessibility. Throughout this chapter, we will delve into the foundational science behind regenerative medicine, explore groundbreaking therapies, and openly discuss the critical challenges that must be addressed to realize its full potential in recalibrating our experience of aging.

The Science of Regeneration

Aging gradually diminishes the body's remarkable ability to repair and regenerate itself. Over time, cells become less efficient, tissues struggle more to recover from injuries, and overall regenerative processes markedly slow down. Three key biological factors drive this decline: cellular senescence, chronic inflammation, and diminished stem cell function. Chapter 3 explores the scientific theories underpinning these mechanisms in greater detail.

Senescent cells no longer serve their original functions effectively; instead, they persist and release inflammatory signals, damaging healthy neighboring tissues. Chronic inflammation further erodes the body's integrity, hastening aging. Additionally, stem cells—nature's vital toolkit for repair and renewal—decline in both number and effectiveness, reducing inherent healing capabilities.

Regenerative medicine directly tackles these fundamental challenges through innovative approaches such as stem cell therapies, gene editing techniques, tissue engineering, and senolytics. These therapeutic strategies replenish depleted cells, correct genetic vulnerabilities, build entirely new tissues and organs, and remove harmful senescent cells. Collectively, these interventions offer remarkable promise to alter and potentially redirect the aging trajectory.

Regenerative medicine reaches its fullest potential when strategically combined with preventive healthcare practices, optimized nutrition, and active lifestyle choices. Integrating these approaches creates a powerful synergy, effectively enhancing lifespan and substantially improving overall quality of life.

Stem Cell Therapies: Unlocking the Body's Regenerative Potential

Central to regenerative medicine are stem cells, uniquely capable of developing into specialized tissues needed to repair damage. They are classified into three main categories: embryonic stem cells (ESCs), adult stem cells, and induced pluripotent stem cells (iPSCs).

Embryonic stem cells, derived from early-stage embryos, have extraordinary versatility but their use raises ethical concerns. Adult stem cells, sourced from bone marrow or adipose (fat) tissues, demonstrate promising results in treatments for orthopedic injuries, cardiovascular conditions, and neurological disorders despite their narrower differentiation range. Induced pluripotent stem cells represent a pioneering solution—adult cells reprogrammed into a highly versatile state, avoiding ethical issues and enabling personalized treatments.

Stem cell therapies are positively influencing numerous medical fields. Orthopedic researchers are exploring treatments to regenerate cartilage, potentially restoring mobility and alleviating pain for arthritis patients. Cardiology studies investigate their capacity to repair heart tissues damaged by heart attacks, aiming to reduce long-term heart failure risks. Neuroscience research focuses on regenerating neurons to potentially mitigate diseases such as Parkinson's and Alzheimer's. Conditions involving vision impairment, like macular degeneration, and pancreatic dysfunction associated with diabetes are also increasingly addressed through regenerative techniques.

However, significant scientific hurdles remain, including immune rejection, uncontrolled cell proliferation, and tumor formation. Researchers are diligently working to overcome these through precision-guided differentiation protocols, advanced biomaterials, and targeted delivery systems. Moreover, integrating cutting-edge technologies like CRISPR gene editing and artificial intelligence-driven personalized treatment protocols promises further breakthroughs, enhancing the effectiveness, accessibility, and affordability of these therapies.

As scientific advances accelerate, stem cell therapies are poised to shape the future of regenerative medicine. Their promise lies not only in repairing what time erodes, but in reawakening the body's innate capacity for renewal—redefining the contours of aging and the possibilities of human repair.

IOULIA HOWARD AND DON HOWARD

Extracellular Vesicles and Exosome Therapy

Stem cell therapy has long been foundational to regenerative medicine, yet recent discoveries have spotlighted a fascinating new frontier: exosomes. These microscopic extracellular vesicles, measuring less than 100 nanometers, act as tiny biological couriers. They carry a sophisticated payload—including proteins, RNA, growth factors, and signaling molecules. This payload orchestrates inflammation regulation, healing acceleration, and regeneration stimulation.

Exosome therapy offers many regenerative benefits similar to traditional stem cell treatments but without introducing living cells. This approach significantly reduces risks such as immune rejection, tumor development, or unintended cellular differentiation. Early research already indicates promising outcomes; exosomes derived from mesenchymal stem cells (MSCs) accelerate tissue repair, provide neuroprotective effects in conditions like strokes and neurodegenerative diseases, and enhance wound healing and skin rejuvenation.

Beyond regenerative medicine, exosomes are opening new therapeutic avenues due to their unique ability to deliver therapeutic agents precisely to targeted tissues. Early-stage investigations suggest their potential role in cancer treatment, facilitating more accurate drug delivery directly to tumor sites. Major obstacles must still be overcome before exosomes can achieve widespread clinical use—including optimizing scalable production methods, defining consistent therapeutic protocols, and developing clear, comprehensive regulatory guidelines.

If researchers successfully address these challenges, exosome therapy could soon represent a powerful, minimally invasive tool, enhancing and amplifying the body's natural healing processes. Such advancements promise broader therapeutic applications across diverse medical conditions. Although the journey ahead requires substantial research, exosome therapy offers genuine hope for reshaping clinical treatments and advancing healthcare.

Regenerating the Human Body: The Future of Tissue Engineering and Bioprinting

Tissue engineering and bioprinting represent groundbreaking advances in regenerative medicine, offering remarkable new possibilities for repairing, replacing, and regenerating human tissues and organs. By seamlessly combining biological insights with innovative bioengineering techniques—such as 3D bioprinting, bioactive scaffolds, and organoid development—these technologies are poised to address critical healthcare challenges, including shortages of donor organs, degenerative diseases, and chronic injuries.

At the heart of tissue engineering is the concept of harnessing the body's innate healing abilities. Scientists utilize biocompatible scaffolds, living cells, and bioactive molecules to craft tissues specifically tailored to individual patients. Today, personalized skin grafts created through this method transform burn care, reducing rejection risks and accelerating healing. Recent innovations even incorporate hair follicles, sweat glands, and pigmentation, significantly improving patient outcomes in reconstructive surgery.

In orthopedics, engineered cartilage offers newfound hope to those living with arthritis or traumatic injuries, potentially delaying or eliminating the need for joint replacement surgeries. By closely replicating natural cartilage, these bioengineered tissues integrate smoothly with existing tissues, offering more lasting relief. Meanwhile, cardiovascular medicine continues to advance bioengineered heart valves and vessels, aiming to enhance durability and reduce complications for patients with heart conditions.

The ultimate goal of tissue engineering—creating fully functional, transplantable organs on-demand—remains an ambitious challenge. While 3D bioprinting allows precise layering of living cells and growth factors, significant advancements are still needed to achieve fully transplantable organs capable of essential functions, such as waste filtration in kidneys, toxin metabolism in livers, or rhythmic beating in hearts. These sophisticated functionalities demand precise cellular organization and careful biochemical coordination, supported by ongoing advances in stem cell research, bioactive growth factors, genetic reprogramming, and bioreactor technology.

Complementing these efforts, organoid research involves creating miniature, self-organizing structures from stem cells. These tiny yet complex organoids mimic the behavior and architecture of actual organs, providing invaluable tools for disease modeling, personalized medicine, and drug testing. Organoids thus offer a fascinating glimpse into the future potential of personalized organ replacements.

Xenotransplantation—the transplantation of genetically modified animal organs into humans—is also progressing rapidly. A landmark achievement in 2022 demonstrated the feasibility of pig-to-human heart transplants, made possible by CRISPR gene-editing techniques that minimize immune rejection. This significant milestone highlights xenotransplantation's potential role in alleviating the chronic shortage of donor organs.

Another promising approach is decellularization, in which donor organs are stripped of cells, leaving behind their natural extracellular matrix. This scaffold can then be repopulated with a recipient's own cells, significantly reducing immune rejection risks and providing a practical route toward personalized organ transplants. Early successes, particularly with heart scaffolds, underscore decellularization's potential as an immediate solution while full organ bioprinting continues to mature.

Despite these exciting developments, substantial hurdles remain before engineered organs become commonplace in clinical medicine. A particularly complex challenge involves creating functional vascular networks within engineered tissues to ensure adequate nutrient and oxygen supply for cell survival. Researchers are actively exploring innovative approaches such as angiogenic biomaterials, microfluidic technologies, and advanced bioreactors to facilitate capillary formation and integration.

Alongside technical advancements, ethical and regulatory considerations must be thoughtfully addressed. Questions surrounding equitable access, clinical safety standards, and manufacturing protocols necessitate careful policymaking and public discourse to ensure these advanced therapies benefit everyone, rather than becoming exclusive to privileged groups.

Together, tissue engineering, bioprinting, decellularization, and xenotransplantation are opening unprecedented avenues in regenerative medicine and organ transplantation. As researchers overcome existing barriers—such as vascularization, functional integration, scalability, and ethical concerns—these technologies are steadily progressing from theoretical possibilities toward real-world applications. Ultimately, regenerative medicine promises not only to revolutionize organ transplantation but also to fundamentally change how we treat disease, extend healthspan, and harness the body's remarkable ability to heal, regenerate, and renew itself.

Bioelectric Medicine: Regenerating Tissues with Electrical Stimulation

Electricity plays a fundamental role in nearly all biological processes—from the rhythmic beating of our hearts to the delicate signaling that allows our neurons to communicate. This invisible force guides our muscles, coordinates our cells, and underlies the complex dance of cellular repair. Recently, a remarkable field known as bioelectric medicine (or electroceuticals) has harnessed this natural phenomenon, using carefully controlled electrical stimulation to encourage tissue regeneration, accelerate healing, and potentially restore function to damaged organs.

One particularly exciting application of bioelectric medicine lies in nerve regeneration. Individuals suffering from spinal cord injuries or neurodegenerative conditions such as Parkinson's disease now have new reasons for hope. By applying targeted electrical stimulation, bioelectric implants have successfully reactivated previously dormant nerve pathways, enabling some patients to regain partial mobility. This achievement marks a profound step forward in neurological rehabilitation. Ongoing research is also exploring how controlled electrical signals might stimulate neuroplasticity—the brain's remarkable ability to reorganize and repair itself—potentially slowing or even halting the progression of debilitating neurodegenerative disorders.

Yet, the transformative potential of bioelectric medicine extends well beyond neurology. Electrical stimulation has also shown promise in activating stem cells, speeding up wound healing, and enhancing overall recovery. For skin injuries, precisely delivered electrical fields replicate the body's own healing signals, directing cells to the injury site and dramatically accelerating recovery. Early studies even suggest that these electrical signals could awaken dormant stem cells. This discovery provides novel avenues to counteract age-related tissue deterioration.

As bioelectric medicine continues to mature, its combination with other innovative regenerative approaches—such as stem cell therapy, tissue engineering, and gene editing—could unlock unprecedented therapeutic opportunities. These complementary strategies, when integrated, may facilitate multifaceted treatments targeting healing at cellular, molecular, and systemic levels. Additionally, the minimally invasive nature of many bioelectric techniques further enhances their attractiveness. Such approaches position bioelectric medicine as a powerful ally in neurological rehabilitation, chronic pain management, and possibly even organ regeneration.

Once a concept seemingly confined to science fiction, the reality of regenerating tissues through electricity is rapidly becoming tangible. Although substantial scientific hurdles remain, the steady progress achieved thus far underscores bioelectric medicine's extraordinary promise. Could the careful application of electrical stimulation soon change the way we understand healing and regeneration?

Ethical and Practical Considerations

As regenerative medicine rapidly advances, it presents exciting scientific opportunities alongside significant ethical, practical, and philosophical questions. Among these, the issue of accessibility is particularly critical. Despite the impressive scientific promise, groundbreaking regenerative therapies often carry prohibitively high costs, potentially restricting their availability to only a select, privileged group. This economic barrier risks exacerbating existing healthcare inequalities by placing essential treatments beyond the reach of many who could greatly benefit. Ensuring equitable access is therefore imperative if regenerative medicine is to fulfill its transformative potential.

Ethical considerations extend further than economics alone. Embryonic stem cell research, genetic modification technologies, and experimental longevity treatments raise profound philosophical dilemmas. Society must thoughtfully weigh the considerable benefits these innovations promise against the associated risks and unintended consequences. To responsibly manage these complexities, comprehensive and transparent regulatory frameworks are essential. Such frameworks not only safeguard patient safety and treatment efficacy but also align scientific progress with broadly shared ethical values. Without clear guidelines, distinguishing genuinely valuable medical breakthroughs from ethically questionable practices could become increasingly difficult.

Public education and open dialogue are also central to fostering societal acceptance and understanding of regenerative medicine. The rapid pace of scientific developments frequently outstrips public awareness, creating the potential for confusion, skepticism, or resistance. Transparent and accessible communication about regenerative medicine—its science, potential benefits, and possible risks—is crucial. Such clarity helps build public trust, facilitating informed discussions and evidence-based policy decisions that support responsible integration of these innovations into healthcare systems.

Moving forward, achieving the right balance among scientific innovation, broad accessibility, and ethical responsibility will be paramount. While regenerative medicine offers an undeniably captivating promise of significantly extending lifespan and improving healthspan, its ultimate success will be measured by how ethically and widely its benefits are shared across society. Achieving this careful equilibrium will determine whether regenerative medicine truly fulfills its remarkable potential to enhance human health and longevity.

The Future of Regenerative Medicine— Pushing Scientific Frontiers

Regenerative medicine is spearheading a fundamental shift in healthcare—from primarily managing symptoms toward genuine biological repair and rejuvenation. Throughout our exploration, we've discovered diverse and innovative scientific approaches. These range from precise stem cell differentiation and exosome-driven cellular communication to sophisticated engineering of complex tissues and organs via advanced bioprinting and novel biomaterials. Additional breakthroughs, including bioelectric medicine, xenotransplantation, and revolutionary gene-editing techniques, further underscore regenerative science's potential to radically redefine human health and longevity.

As research continues to progress, scientists face essential technical challenges. Achieving precise cellular control, ensuring immune compatibility, developing functional vascular systems for engineered tissues, and guaranteeing the seamless integration of bioengineered treatments within the human body are among the hurdles researchers must overcome. Concurrently, ethical issues—such as responsible genetic modification, sourcing stem cells ethically, and ensuring equitable access to treatments—require ongoing, careful consideration.

Regenerative medicine presents a hopeful scientific vision. It aims not just to extend human lifespan, but also to significantly enhance quality of life. By continuously advancing the boundaries of biology, engineering, and medical technology—while remaining mindful of ethical imperatives—regenerative medicine promises a future in which enhanced physical capacity, sustained well-being, and greater adaptive strength become accessible realities for everyone.

CHAPTER 20

Gene Therapy: Editing the Future of Aging

"There is nothing in a caterpillar that tells you it's going to be a butterfly."
—R. BUCKMINSTER FULLER

Gene therapy—the intricate science of rewriting biology's blueprint to treat or prevent disease—is challenging conventional views of aging and illness. By engaging directly with DNA, life's foundational blueprint, scientists are exploring extraordinary opportunities to slow and perhaps even reverse aging. In this chapter, we navigate the complex yet captivating world of gene therapy, highlighting current breakthroughs and uncovering its growing promise to extend lifespan and augment quality of life.

Gene Therapy and the Revolutionary Promise of CRISPR

Among the most remarkable advancements in gene therapy is the development of CRISPR technology. Initially discovered as a natural immune defense mechanism in bacteria, CRISPR (Clustered Regularly Interspaced Short Palindromic Repeats) has been adeptly adapted by researchers for precise DNA editing. CRISPR carefully locates and alters specific genetic targets, enabling corrections to harmful mutations, repair of genetic defects, and the introduction of beneficial traits. This level of accuracy significantly enhances our ability to address the complex mechanisms underlying aging.

Already, scientists are leveraging CRISPR's precision to confront age-related diseases at their genetic origins. For instance, precisely targeting genes such as APP and PSEN1—which are involved in the formation of amyloid plaques characteristic of Alzheimer's disease—may offer preventive strategies against its neurodegeneration, potentially safeguarding cognitive health long before symptoms emerge. Similarly, CRISPR-based therapies aimed at correcting genetic factors responsible for age-related macular degeneration could protect vision over time. In cardiovascular health, editing the PCSK9 gene has demonstrated striking effectiveness in reducing cholesterol, greatly lowering the risk of heart disease—a leading contributor to aging-related mortality.

Advances like base editing and prime editing further expand CRISPR's potential by enabling precise modifications to single DNA bases, significantly reducing unintended genetic alterations. Additionally, integrating CRISPR with artificial intelligence refines gene-editing accuracy and target selection, fostering cautious yet tangible optimism within longevity research.

Despite its promise, CRISPR presents important challenges, including concerns about unintended genetic changes and ethical considerations surrounding germline editing—alterations inheritable by future generations. These issues require careful oversight and ongoing public discussion. Yet, as CRISPR technology evolves alongside other scientific innovations, it increasingly stands at the forefront of efforts to rewrite the biological story of aging.

Reprogramming Aging: Broader Gene Therapy Approaches

While CRISPR often captures the spotlight, numerous other gene therapy approaches hold substantial promise for addressing aging. Methods such as epigenetic reprogramming and mitochondrial restoration complement CRISPR's precision, collectively expanding the horizon of possibilities to enhance health and extend lifespan. Among these, epigenetic reprogramming stands out, exemplified by techniques employing Yamanaka factors—a set of proteins capable of returning mature cells to a youthful, stem-cell-like state. Rather than directly altering DNA, these methods carefully reset cellular age by adjusting gene-expression patterns. The promise here is extraordinary, though achieving it requires careful, tightly regulated steps to avoid potential risks.

Synthetic biology and immune rejuvenation represent additional dimensions of gene therapy's potential. Synthetic biology creatively engineers genetic pathways to optimize metabolism, encourage tissue regeneration, and fortify cellular resilience. Meanwhile, immune rejuvenation strategies aim to enhance the clearance of senescent cells, aging cells known to promote chronic inflammation and tissue deterioration, thereby restoring physiological balance.

Still, important hurdles must be overcome, particularly regarding the precise delivery of genetic therapies, long-term safety assurances, and practical cost considerations. Nevertheless, ongoing clinical research continues to steadily advance these sophisticated approaches from theory into clinical reality. Collectively, these broader gene therapy strategies, in combination with CRISPR innovations, challenge our long-held assumptions about aging. Rather than an unavoidable decline, could aging become a manageable—even reversible—condition? The science unfolding today suggests such a remarkable possibility.

Beyond Repair: Boosting Longevity Genes

Advances in gene therapy are steadily shifting from repairing existing damage toward proactively nurturing the body's intrinsic capacity for longevity. Rather than simply correcting genetic defects after they arise, emerging therapies now aim to enhance natural genetic pathways that sustain long-term health, resilience, and extended lifespan.

A particularly exciting frontier in longevity science involves strategically influencing genetic pathways that counteract aging and strengthen cellular resilience. By amplifying the function of longevity-associated genes like FOXO3 and SIRT6, researchers are discovering new ways to stimulate intrinsic mechanisms for DNA repair, enhance cellular defenses against stress, and maintain metabolic equilibrium—all foundational elements in slowing the pace of biological aging. Equally compelling is the activation of the TERT gene, which produces the enzyme telomerase, essential for preserving the integrity of telomeres and sustaining cellular renewal over time. As our understanding deepens, novel interventions—from targeted lifestyle adjustments to pharmacological and genetic therapies—are emerging, creating fresh possibilities for extending lifespan while enhancing its quality.

Additionally, researchers are investigating genetic interventions that target critical pathways in the aging process. Fine-tuning the activity of the NRF2 gene, a key regulator of the body's antioxidant defenses, offers potential protection against oxidative stress, a fundamental contributor to cellular aging. Likewise, carefully modulating NF-κB, a central regulator of inflammation, may reduce chronic inflammation (known as "inflammaging"), which significantly impacts aging-related decline.

By moving from reactive repairs to proactive genetic enhancements, gene therapy is redefining possibilities for human longevity. These innovative efforts represent a major advancement in aging science, opening new avenues to preserve youthful function and vitality by thoughtfully leveraging the body's own genetic resources.

Navigating the Challenges: Scientific, Ethical, and Societal Considerations

Gene therapy holds immense promise for extending human longevity. Yet alongside this potential lies a complex landscape filled with scientific, ethical, and social hurdles. Modifying our genetic makeup presents transformative opportunities but also unprecedented responsibility. Ensuring lifespan-enhancing efforts simplify rather than complicate human existence requires thoughtful oversight.

Precision remains one of gene therapy's greatest scientific challenges. CRISPR technology has demonstrated impressive accuracy in genetic editing, but significant concerns persist regarding unintended, off-target effects. Such accidental genetic alterations could lead to instability or harmful mutations, potentially elevating cancer risks. Newer editing techniques, like base editing and prime editing, have improved precision, yet flawless control remains elusive. As gene therapy moves beyond treating specific diseases toward broadly addressing aging, the demand for absolute precision intensifies.

Ethical complexities compound these technical difficulties. Germline editing, which could impact future generations, raises profound moral dilemmas even if proven safe. Should society allow modifications to humanity's genetic legacy? Who decides which traits warrant enhancement? How do we differentiate medical interventions clearly from enhancements of human capabilities? Such questions challenge our moral reasoning as deeply as our scientific capacities.

Societal consequences of gene therapy advancements will also be substantial. Delaying or reversing aging could significantly reshape healthcare, workforce structures, economic systems, and family dynamics. Imagine retaining youthful strength and energy well into advanced age. How might retirement and career paths change? Could longer lifespans provoke unforeseen political or social issues, or might they instead unlock extraordinary human potential?

Fair access to these therapies is vital. Should gene therapies primarily benefit the wealthy, society could see the emergence of a genetically privileged class. Integrating gene therapies fairly within public healthcare systems is essential to prevent widening social inequalities.

Balancing scientific innovation, rigorous regulation, and inclusive dialogue is key to achieving an egalitarian society. Extending lifespan alone is insufficient; ensuring these benefits are shared equally is paramount. The path we choose—toward equitable innovation or greater disparity—depends largely upon the balance struck between progress and responsibility.

The Future of Gene Therapy and Aging: What's Coming Next?

The future of gene therapy in longevity science is poised at the threshold of extraordinary possibilities, driven by innovations that vastly exceed our current capabilities. Among the most promising developments is multiplexed gene editing—a revolutionary technique enabling simultaneous modification of multiple genetic targets, a substantial leap beyond traditional single-gene approaches. A striking example of this advanced technology is MAGESTIC (Multiplexed Accurate Genome Editing with Short, Trackable, Integrated Cellular Barcodes), which not only precisely edits multiple genes in parallel but also allows researchers to meticulously track and evaluate each genetic alteration. Imagine, for instance, a scenario where scientists could concurrently enhance DNA repair efficiency, optimize metabolic pathways, and fortify cells against stress—all within a single integrated intervention. Such a multidimensional approach promises to address the complexities of aging in ways previously unattainable, ushering in a new era of possibility for extending and enriching human life.

Additionally, integrating gene editing with advanced stem cell therapies could open new avenues in regenerative medicine. Enhancing stem cells prior to transplantation may greatly increase their potential for regeneration, enabling the reversal of degenerative conditions throughout entire organ systems. Coupled with emerging epigenetic reprogramming techniques, this holistic approach offers promising possibilities for comprehensive cellular rejuvenation and systemic restoration.

Artificial intelligence is also poised to significantly enhance gene therapy outcomes. By analyzing extensive datasets, AI-powered computational models enable personalized genetic interventions, tailored precisely to individual needs. This targeted approach ensures higher safety, improved efficacy, and greater predictability in therapeutic results.

Despite these remarkable innovations, essential questions surrounding long-term safety, ethical considerations, and clinical practicality must still be thoroughly addressed. Nevertheless, as research advances, gene therapy steadily transforms our understanding of aging—from an inevitable decline to a scientifically manageable, modifiable condition.

Final Thoughts: The Age of Genetic Longevity

Gene therapy stands poised at the forefront of a scientific revolution, ripe with possibilities that researchers have only just begun to explore. This rapidly evolving field goes beyond changing medicine—it dismantles old paradigms about aging, disease prevention, and human potential. By intervening directly at the genetic level, scientists are now able to influence previously immutable aspects of biology, opening doors to innovations once considered purely theoretical.

Each new breakthrough in gene therapy—whether through cellular reprogramming, targeted genetic editing, or the regeneration of tissues—brings unprecedented clarity to the complexities of aging and cellular health. These discoveries not only illuminate how aging occurs at the most fundamental level but also introduce tangible opportunities to counteract, delay, or even reverse processes long assumed inevitable.

Beyond longevity, gene therapy offers the possibility of altering the trajectory of chronic diseases and age-related disorders. Conditions once accepted as permanent or incurable, such as certain genetic disorders, neurodegenerative diseases, and chronic metabolic conditions, are increasingly becoming targets of genetic intervention. Consequently, gene therapy is gradually transforming from a niche experimental tool into a mainstream therapeutic strategy.

Yet, this exciting frontier also brings ethical complexities and practical challenges. The implications of altering human genetics require careful navigation, thoughtful regulation, and broad societal discourse. Questions around equitable access, long-term safety, unintended genetic consequences, and ethical boundaries will undoubtedly accompany gene therapy's ascent into widespread clinical use.

Despite these challenges, the promise of gene therapy remains overwhelmingly positive. We are now witnessing the emergence of a remarkable scientific era, where genetic knowledge empowers us not only to extend lifespan but also to reimagine the experience of aging. Humanity stands on the cusp of a future where genetic longevity becomes less a dream and more a tangible reality, marking the beginning of an extraordinary journey whose most transformative discoveries still lie ahead.

CHAPTER 21

Technology and Longevity: Innovations Shaping Our Healthspan

"Any sufficiently advanced technology is indistinguishable from magic."
—ARTHUR C. CLARKE

Modern technology is rapidly advancing our understanding of health and aging, offering powerful tools that not only promise to extend lifespan but also enhance healthspan. Breakthroughs in artificial intelligence, gene editing, nanotechnology, and robotics are transforming medical treatment, opening new frontiers in human wellness. Innovations once considered the stuff of science fiction are now on the brink of revolutionize how we repair, regenerate, and augment the human body in ways previously thought impossible.

Advances such as real-time health monitoring through wearable devices and CRISPR's ability to rewrite genetic blueprints are disrupting our approach to longevity. As the lines between prevention and enhancement become increasingly blurred, this chapter delves into the transformative technologies that are shaping the future of medicine. It explores their vast potential, while also examining the ethical dilemmas, logistical challenges, and societal implications that accompany their integration into everyday life.

IOULIA HOWARD AND DON HOWARD

Wearable Technology: A New Era of Health Monitoring and Innovation

Wearable technology is changing the way personal health is managed, evolving from basic fitness trackers into advanced devices offering real-time, actionable insights. Smartwatches, fitness bands, and health rings now accurately monitor essential health metrics such as heart rate, sleep quality, physical activity, and stress resilience. Beyond these fundamental functions, sophisticated sensors can measure additional indicators including hydration levels, oxygen saturation (SpO_2), changes in skin temperature, and minute electrodermal signals reflecting stress responses. Particularly significant is the integration of electrocardiogram (ECG) technology, allowing users to instantly record cardiac activity, identify irregular heart rhythms like atrial fibrillation, and rapidly share vital information with healthcare providers—enabling prompt and potentially life-saving interventions.

But the evolution doesn't stop here. Wearable technology continues to evolve rapidly, promising deeper physiological insights and advanced, non-invasive diagnostic capabilities. Think of cuff-free blood pressure monitors utilizing optical or bioimpedance sensors for continuous tracking, or hydration sensors capable of interpreting bioelectric signals and sweat chemistry to optimize fluid intake precisely when needed. Meanwhile, continuous glucose monitors (CGMs)—once exclusively used in diabetic care—are rapidly finding mainstream adoption, guiding personalized dietary choices and metabolic management. Researchers are also making strides toward non-invasive glucose monitoring, potentially eliminating the need for uncomfortable procedures altogether.

Further advancements point toward an extraordinary role for wearables in disease prevention and early diagnosis. Emerging devices capable of detecting molecular biomarkers indicative of early-stage cancers hold the potential to transform prognosis and significantly enhance treatment outcomes. Beyond wrist-based gadgets, the field now encompasses innovative smart fabrics embedded unobtrusively with biosensors that effortlessly track vital signs, posture, hydration, and stress levels. Additionally, implantable biosensors placed discreetly beneath the skin continuously monitor critical parameters such as glucose, heart function, and hormonal fluctuations, enabling highly individualized health management attuned precisely to personal biological rhythms.

Artificial intelligence (AI) is positioned to further elevate wearable technology's potential. AI-driven algorithms can sift through extensive datasets from wearables, identifying subtle physiological shifts, predicting health risks before they become symptomatic, and recommending personalized interventions. Integrating wearable technology with electronic health records (EHRs) could enhance healthcare connectivity, enabling providers instant access to patients' real-time health data, facilitating quicker diagnoses and more effective medical responses.

Wearable technology's progress signals a definitive shift from passive monitoring to active, personalized health management. With comprehensive data readily available, predictive insights guiding their choices, and seamless integration into broader healthcare systems, users stand at the threshold of a new era in preventive medicine—one defined by precision, personalization, and proactive engagement in their own well-being.

Foundational Innovations: CRISPR and Bioprinting in the Future of Longevity

In earlier chapters, we explored two remarkable technological breakthroughs significantly altering our understanding of aging and healthcare. First, we examined CRISPR, the revolutionary gene-editing tool impacting various fields from agriculture to personalized medicine. With unprecedented precision, CRISPR offers the potential to treat, prevent, and possibly even reverse certain aspects of aging at the genetic level.

We also delved into tissue engineering and bioprinting, highlighting how the integration of biological sciences and advanced engineering is transforming regenerative medicine. These innovative techniques not only enable tissue repair but also pave the way toward creating fully functional, personalized organs. Such advancements promise significant improvements in managing age-related degeneration and organ failure, enhancing overall quality of life.

Moving forward, these insights into CRISPR, tissue engineering, and bioprinting provide essential context for understanding the broader landscape of technological innovations rapidly refashioning aging and healthcare.

Nanotechnology in Medicine

Nanotechnology is introducing a new era of precision medicine, allowing treatments to be meticulously tailored at the cellular and molecular levels. This groundbreaking approach promises more accurate interventions, which will alter healthcare by changing diagnostics, drug delivery, and regenerative medicine in ways previously unimaginable.

At the forefront of this revolution are nanobots—tiny, engineered machines capable of navigating the body's complex biological pathways with exceptional accuracy. These nanoscale devices may one day deliver therapies directly to diseased cells, minimizing side effects and boosting treatment effectiveness. Additionally, nanobots could perform diverse therapeutic tasks, including repairing damaged DNA, clearing blocked arteries, or dissolving harmful protein plaques associated with neurodegenerative diseases like Alzheimer's. Although much of this potential remains theoretical, steady advancements in research continue to bring these futuristic applications closer to reality.

Meanwhile, nanosensors are ushering in a new era of early disease detection by identifying minute biomarkers within blood or tissue samples. This heightened sensitivity enables the diagnosis of conditions like cancer and cardiovascular diseases long before noticeable symptoms appear. Early identification in this way can significantly enhance treatment outcomes and patient well-being.

As research advances, nanotechnology is emerging as one of modern medicine's most promising frontiers, addressing diseases directly at their molecular origins. Each innovation moves us closer to breakthroughs capable of significantly extending healthspan and enhancing quality of life. However, considerable refinement, rigorous research, and comprehensive clinical validation remain essential steps before these technologies can achieve widespread clinical adoption.

Digital Twin Technology: The Future of Precision Healthcare and Longevity

Digital twin technology has the potential to reimagine healthcare by evolving traditional medical records into dynamic, real-time simulations of an individual's unique biological systems. Unlike conventional health files—which typically capture static snapshots of past conditions—digital twins continuously integrate data from wearable devices, medical imaging, genetic sequencing, and lifestyle inputs. This dynamic representation offers clinicians and patients alike a continuously updated, real-time perspective on health, enabling more personalized and proactive care.

Central to this evolution are artificial intelligence (AI) and machine learning (ML). These technologies analyze vast, intricate health data, allowing digital twins to simulate organ functions, metabolic processes, and cellular behaviors with remarkable precision. These virtual models enable healthcare providers and researchers to explore and virtually test interventions—such as medication adjustments, dietary optimizations, or novel gene therapies—before applying them in real-world scenarios. Although still emerging, these predictive capabilities offer tremendous potential to enhance treatment safety, improve efficacy, and minimize adverse reactions.

Beyond immediate medical applications, digital twin technology is opening new frontiers in longevity research. Researchers use these sophisticated simulations to investigate long-term outcomes of longevity-focused strategies such as caloric restriction, senolytic therapies, and epigenetic reprogramming. By modeling the effects of these interventions on metabolism, immune response, and overall healthspan, digital twins significantly accelerate the development of targeted, effective anti-aging treatments. In pharmacology, this technology helps tailor drug therapies to individual genetic profiles, maximizing therapeutic benefits and minimizing risks.

Digital twins also empower people to take greater control of their personal health. Instead of relying on generalized health advice, each person can access customized recommendations based on real-time data that captures their body's unique responses to exercise, diet, and environmental factors. Moving beyond the traditional trial-and-error healthcare model, digital twin technology provides precise, personalized guidance tailored to meet individual health goals.

However, significant challenges remain. Constructing reliable digital twins requires sophisticated algorithms that accurately represent human biology's complexity. Privacy and data security are paramount concerns, given the sensitive nature of personal health information. Equitable access to this transformative technology is equally vital; ensuring these benefits reach everyone, regardless of socioeconomic status, is essential to prevent deepening healthcare disparities.

Despite these challenges, digital twins hold immense potential. Imagine a future where each person has a dynamic, virtual counterpart continually adapting to offer personalized insights for disease prevention, optimized treatments, and enhanced physical and cognitive well-being. By refining therapies, predicting diseases before onset, and improving healthspan, digital twin technology may materially alter our approach to healthcare—crafting a future where health decisions are guided by our virtual counterparts.

Robotics in Practice—Transforming Surgery and Rehabilitation

The integration of advanced robotics into medical practice is igniting innovation in surgical care and rehabilitation, converting once-complex procedures into more precise, efficient, and patient-friendly experiences. These systems are no longer speculative tools of the future—they are actively moulding healthcare in the present.

In surgery, platforms like the da Vinci Surgical System have established a new standard for minimally invasive procedures. With articulated robotic arms controlled by the surgeon via a console, these systems deliver high-definition, three-dimensional visualization and unmatched dexterity. By filtering out hand tremors and enabling microscale movements, robotic systems facilitate greater precision in complex procedures such as prostatectomies, cardiac valve repairs, and tumor resections. Clinical studies consistently show improved outcomes, including smaller incisions, reduced blood loss, shorter hospital stays, and faster recovery times, when compared to traditional open surgery.

Robotic technologies are also advancing physical rehabilitation. Wearable exoskeletons, developed by companies like ReWalk Robotics and Ekso Bionics, provide powered assistance to individuals with impaired mobility due to spinal cord injuries, strokes, or neurodegenerative disorders. These devices enable users to stand, walk, and perform daily activities with greater independence, while also supporting musculoskeletal health by improving muscle strength, circulation, and bone density. In clinical settings, robotic gait-training platforms such as the Lokomat deliver feedback-driven, repetitive motion therapy tailored to each patient's capacity. This approach enhances neuroplasticity and accelerates motor recovery beyond the limits of conventional therapies.

These robotic systems demonstrate that technological augmentation can restore function, reduce risk, and improve quality of life—especially when integrated into personalized care strategies. As the field evolves, their role in medicine will only deepen, particularly as they interface with intelligent systems capable of learning and adapting to patient needs.

Beyond Mechanics—Bioelectronics and the Future of Functional Medicine

Building upon the mechanical precision of robotics, bioelectronics harnesses the body's natural electrical signaling to restore physiological function. It moves beyond traditional drug-based approaches, directly targeting neural pathways involved in disease. For example, vagus nerve stimulation (VNS), initially approved for epilepsy and treatment-resistant depression, now shows potential for controlling chronic inflammation—a critical factor in aging and age-related illnesses. Similarly, established bioelectronic interventions like pacemakers, defibrillators, and deep brain stimulators have demonstrated how precise electrical modulation can effectively treat conditions such as arrhythmias, Parkinson's disease, and chronic pain.

Yet bioelectronics is venturing further. Peripheral nerve stimulators, currently in development, offer hope for restoring motor control, autonomic regulation, and sensory perception after spinal cord injuries or nerve damage. Rather than mechanically replacing lost functions, these cutting-edge devices reawaken dormant neural pathways, tapping into the body's innate capacity for repair.

Expanding the Frontiers of Longevity Technology

What happens when robotics, bioelectronics, and artificial intelligence (AI) combine forces? The result is a wave of healthcare innovation pioneering a new direction in our approach to longevity. AI-enhanced bioelectronic implants dynamically optimize nerve stimulation, delivering personalized and adaptive treatments. At the same time, robotic rehabilitation systems intelligently adjust therapies in real-time, significantly boosting therapeutic effectiveness. Even preventive healthcare benefits from wearable bioelectronic devices that continuously monitor vital physiological markers—heart rate variability, inflammation levels, and neural activity—catching early indicators of aging well before symptoms become apparent.

For aging populations, robotics will soon become a fundamental part of daily life, seamlessly facilitating everyday tasks, improving mobility, and encouraging active lifestyles. Meanwhile, augmented reality (AR) and virtual reality (VR)—once primarily tools for entertainment—are expanding into essential roles in diagnostics, medical training, rehabilitation, and mental healthcare, enriching life experiences.

Collectively, these technologies do far more than simply manage disease. They support longevity, empowering older adults to maintain their independence and engagement throughout their lifespans. With AI-driven diagnostics, robotic-assisted therapies, and sophisticated bioelectronic implants, medicine is shifting toward a predictive, personalized model, significantly recasting our expectations of health and aging.

Virtual and Augmented Reality: Transforming Pain Management, Mental Health, Cognitive Function, and Rehabilitation

Virtual reality (VR) immerses users completely into digital, simulated worlds, while augmented reality (AR) enriches real-world environments by seamlessly overlaying digital elements onto physical surroundings.

These groundbreaking technologies are ushering in a new era of healthcare and wellness, offering immersive solutions across diverse medical fields. Virtual reality (VR), with its vivid and engaging experiences, has shown remarkable effectiveness in managing chronic pain, supporting mental health, and enhancing cognitive function. Patients coping with conditions such as fibromyalgia or recovering from surgery can experience meaningful relief by stepping into tranquil virtual landscapes—peaceful beaches, lush forests, or serene underwater scenes—that gently shift attention away from discomfort.

In mental health settings, VR is advancing exposure therapy. Individuals facing PTSD, social anxiety, or related challenges can safely confront and reprocess distressing experiences within controlled, therapeutic simulations. Additionally, VR-based cognitive exercises actively stimulate memory, enhance problem-solving skills, and sharpen attention, playing a vital role in slowing cognitive decline and strengthening neural connections, particularly valuable in aging populations.

AR, though less immersive, offers equally significant contributions to cognitive support and rehabilitation. By integrating real-time digital cues, AR supports older adults in memory training, spatial awareness, and performing daily tasks independently. Within physical rehabilitation, AR provides immediate, practical feedback on posture, alignment, and movement quality—crucial for stroke survivors and those recovering from injuries. This technology effectively retrains motor skills and promotes proper movement patterns.

VR pushes rehabilitation even further by creating dynamic, realistic environments that replicate everyday activities. Stroke survivors and injury patients can safely practice real-life tasks—reaching, grasping, navigating—in risk-free simulated scenarios. By incorporating elements of gamification and personalized progress tracking, VR fosters motivation, sustained participation, and quicker recovery outcomes.

Together, these immersive technologies represent a paradigm-shifting advance in healthcare. They deliver personalized, engaging therapies that markedly enhance pain relief, mental well-being, cognitive vitality, and physical rehabilitation, thereby enriching patient experiences and substantially improving quality of life.

Fitness and Longevity: Making Exercise Engaging and Effective

Virtual and augmented reality are changing the way we approach fitness and exercise, introducing dynamic, interactive experiences that make physical health both engaging and fun. Imagine stepping into a virtual world where you can box, dance, scale mountains, or explore breathtaking new environments—all while getting a full-body workout. Platforms like Supernatural and FitXR have elevated exercise into an engaging, game-like experience, delivering a level of motivation and consistency often missing from traditional workouts.

In contrast, augmented reality (AR) fitness applications provide real-time coaching that overlays helpful cues directly into your field of vision. Whether you're practicing yoga, weightlifting, or Pilates, AR ensures you maintain proper posture and technique, reducing the risk of injury while improving performance. For older adults, AR-guided exercises become even more invaluable, focusing on crucial elements such as balance, mobility, and strength training—key factors for fall prevention and maintaining long-term physical resilience.

Advancing Medical Training and Surgical Precision

The integration of virtual reality (VR) and augmented reality (AR) is remapping the landscape of medical education and surgical training. VR provides healthcare professionals the opportunity to practice complex procedures in highly realistic, risk-free environments. These simulations allow practitioners to refine their skills without involving live patients, significantly enhancing their readiness for real-world scenarios. From basic diagnostic training to intricate surgical rehearsals, VR is rapidly becoming a vital tool in the cultivation of medical expertise.

Meanwhile, AR is enhancing real-world medical practices by providing surgeons with real-time data and visual aids. During surgery, AR systems overlay critical anatomical structures directly onto a surgeon's view, improving precision and minimizing the risk of complications. AR is also proving invaluable in diagnostics, helping physicians interpret medical images with greater accuracy, ultimately leading to more effective treatment plans.

The Age of Intelligent Longevity

The future of longevity is no longer just a distant possibility—it is coalescing from the convergence of rapidly advancing technologies. Innovations in bioelectronics, nanotechnology, gene editing, immersive digital health solutions, and artificial intelligence (explored in detail in the next chapter) are progressing at an extraordinary pace, each accelerating the development of the others. Together, they offer unprecedented opportunities to better understand, manage, and potentially slow the aging process.

In the coming decade, health monitoring will go far beyond today's wearable devices. Ponder a future in which real-time physiological data integrates seamlessly with advanced diagnostic platforms, digital twin simulations, and personalized gene therapies. This interconnected system could shift healthcare from a reactive, illness-driven model to one focused on prevention, prediction, and continuous optimization of biological function. At the same time, regenerative medicine is advancing rapidly. Bioprinted organs, stem cell rejuvenation, and cellular reprogramming are emerging as viable solutions for repairing and revitalizing aging tissues. These developments not only promise significant gains in lifespan and healthspan but also mark a fundamental transition toward proactive, personalized care—allowing people to age with strength, independence, and preserved quality of life.

Naturally, these innovations bring complex challenges. As lifespans and periods of good health extend, societies must adapt to shifting demographic patterns and evolving roles. Ethical considerations surrounding gene editing, intelligent health systems, and human enhancement demand thoughtful regulation and responsible integration. The future of longevity will not be defined solely by scientific breakthroughs, but by how wisely and equitably they are applied.

Looking ahead, emerging technologies continue to deepen our understanding of aging, offering the potential not only to extend life but to enhance its quality at every stage. With sustained progress, we are approaching a future in which well-being, autonomy, and resilience can be preserved well into later life. In this unfolding era, longevity is no longer an aspiration alone—it is becoming a matter of deliberate design, supported by science, guided by purpose, and shaped by innovation.

CHAPTER 22

Artificial Intelligence in Health and Aging: Smarter, Longer Lives

"The only way to discover the limits of the possible is to go beyond them into the impossible."
—ARTHUR C. CLARKE

Historically, medicine has treated aging-related conditions like waiting until the storm is raging before seeking shelter—intervening only after symptoms intensify and complications become entrenched, often overlooking early warnings that could safeguard lifelong health. Today, artificial intelligence (AI)—a rapidly advancing field enabling machines to mimic human cognitive processes—is fundamentally altering this approach. But what exactly is AI, and why is it revolutionary? At its core, AI employs sophisticated techniques such as machine learning, in which algorithms analyze extensive datasets to recognize complex patterns, continually improving their accuracy with experience. Within machine learning, deep learning stands out as particularly powerful, using neural networks—computational structures inspired by the human brain, composed of interconnected nodes or "neurons"—to detect subtle relationships hidden within data. By harnessing these capabilities, AI facilitates early disease detection, personalized treatments, and preventive healthcare strategies.

Precision Foresight: AI's Role in Personalized Healthcare

AI predictive analytics integrate diverse data sources such as genetic profiles, metabolic markers, wearable device metrics, medical imaging, and real-time electronic health records, enhancing the early detection of aging-related illnesses like cancer, cardiovascular disease, and neurodegenerative disorders. For example, traditional medical imaging relies heavily on human interpretation, which can be limited by fatigue or variability. AI-enhanced imaging systems surpass these limitations, empowering clinicians to identify minute abnormalities rapidly and accurately. Similarly, AI-powered histopathology enriches microscopic tissue analysis, bolstering human judgment and diagnostic precision.

Innovative methods like AI-driven liquid biopsies further demonstrate this potential by non-invasively detecting biomarkers in bodily fluids, allowing continuous monitoring of molecular changes linked to various health conditions. AI also impacts genetic diagnostics through techniques such as polygenic risk scoring (PRS), which simultaneously evaluates numerous genetic variants to predict susceptibility to diseases like Alzheimer's and metabolic disorders. While highly promising, these tools require integration with traditional clinical assessments to maximize effectiveness.

Another frontier is digital twin technology, in which AI constructs personalized virtual models simulating an individual's biological responses to diet, exercise, medications, and treatments. As this technology advances from experimental to clinical use, ongoing research will clarify how precisely these virtual models align with actual patient outcomes, opening new possibilities for highly individualized medical care.

On a broader scale, AI significantly strengthens global health surveillance by integrating diverse information—from hospital records and wearable devices to satellite imagery and environmental sensors. During global health crises like the COVID-19 pandemic, AI effectively tracked viral spread, monitored mutations, and guided resource distribution. Nonetheless, challenges persist, including addressing data biases, ensuring algorithm fairness, safeguarding privacy, and promoting equitable healthcare access.

Ultimately, AI's potential extends far beyond simply prolonging lifespan; it prioritizes healthspan, the period characterized by robust physical and cognitive function. By accurately predicting disease risks and enabling customized interventions, AI empowers healthcare providers to significantly enhance patient well-being and long-term health outcomes. Realizing this vision will depend on ongoing advancements in data management, healthcare infrastructure, and ethical guidelines—firmly establishing AI as a cornerstone of healthcare's proactive, personalized future.

From Molecule to Medicine: How AI is Reshaping Drug Discovery

Developing new pharmaceuticals has historically been an arduous, uncertain process, with many promising drugs failing due to unforeseen toxicity or limited effectiveness—setbacks particularly detrimental in longevity research. Artificial intelligence (AI) is rewriting the rules of drug discovery by rapidly and accurately screening vast chemical libraries, predicting molecular interactions with biological targets, and accelerating the identification of promising drug candidates. Although AI's predictions remain probabilistic, laboratory validation continues to be essential for confirming biochemical activity, pharmacodynamics (drug effects on the body), and safety before progressing to clinical trials.

AI also excels at drug repurposing—finding new therapeutic applications for existing medications. Drugs like metformin, rapamycin, and senolytics, initially developed for diabetes, cancer, or immune disorders, are now investigated for anti-aging potential. AI's capacity to analyze large-scale biomedical data swiftly identifies previously unrecognized therapeutic possibilities, creating new research directions that may materially influence clinical practice upon empirical validation.

Clinical trials, typically the most costly and time-consuming stage of drug development, benefit from AI's innovations. By meticulously analyzing medical histories, genetic profiles, and biomarkers, AI improves participant selection, reduces dropout rates, and manages variability in patient responses. Machine learning models further refine trial designs by predicting side effects, optimal dosages, and potential patient reactions. As AI applications expand, robust regulatory oversight, ethical standards, participant diversity, and safety considerations will remain crucial to fully realize its transformative potential in clinical research.

In synthetic biology, AI showcases its innovative capacity by designing novel biological systems and molecules targeting fundamental aging mechanisms, such as mitochondrial function, cellular senescence, and autophagy. Although currently confined to early-stage research, these AI-generated molecules hold substantial promise for future breakthroughs.

Precision Aging: Harnessing AI to Unlock Personalized Biomarkers and Targeted Health Strategies

Aging is a deeply personal process shaped by molecular changes, genetic variations, and metabolic complexities. While chronological age simply measures the passage of time, biological age more accurately reflects a person's physiological state, capturing cellular resilience and environmental factors. But how can we unravel such complexity? Artificial intelligence (AI) provides powerful tools, decoding aging by analyzing extensive biological data—including genomic, metabolic, and proteomic markers, alongside clinical tests, imaging, microbiome profiles, and wearable metrics. The result is sophisticated biomarkers that offer real-time, individualized health insights.

One impactful example involves refining epigenetic clocks—tools estimating biological age by analyzing DNA methylation patterns. AI algorithms pinpoint critical methylation markers, significantly enhancing predictive accuracy. Platforms such as Deep Longevity, Gero.ai, and Horvath's Epigenetic Clock use these innovations to predict aging trajectories and deliver precise biological-age assessments, revealing novel insights into aging mechanisms.

AI further illuminates aging's biochemical foundations through detailed metabolic and proteomic studies. These analyses identify potential therapeutic targets and early indicators of diseases like neurodegeneration and cancer. Simultaneously, AI-enhanced wearable technologies continuously track physiological signals—such as glucose levels, heart rhythms, and sleep patterns—to detect subtle signs of inflammation, circadian disruption, or autonomic dysfunction, complementing clinical assessments and enabling proactive care.

AI heralds a new era of longevity interventions precisely tailored to individual biology. Realizing these innovations fully requires rigorous validation, thoughtful clinical integration, and strong ethical frameworks, ensuring they enhance—rather than replace—established medical practices. As AI continues to accelerate longevity research, comprehensive long-term studies will confirm the sustained impact of these interventions on health outcomes and lifespan extension.

From Reprogramming to Repair: AI's Role in Regenerative Medicine

As we age, our bodies gradually lose their remarkable ability to regenerate tissues, much like a house losing structural integrity over time. This deterioration weakens vital organs and increases susceptibility to conditions such as osteoarthritis, cardiovascular disease, and neurodegenerative disorders, creating an urgent need for effective regenerative therapies. Regenerative medicine, covered extensively in a previous chapter, addresses these challenges by reversing biological damage and restoring tissue functionality—a process now significantly accelerated by artificial intelligence (AI). From stem cell therapies to advanced tissue engineering, AI is charting new frontiers in longevity science.

Stem cell therapy offers a clear illustration of AI's game-changing impact. Historically, guiding stem cells to form specific tissues has proven challenging. AI addresses this challenge by optimizing differentiation protocols through detailed biological analyses, enhancing therapeutic effectiveness and minimizing risks such as uncontrolled growth or immune rejection.

AI also accelerates cellular reprogramming, converting mature cells into youthful, pluripotent forms capable of generating various cell types. By identifying optimal combinations of transcription factors—proteins regulating gene activity and cell behavior—AI fine-tunes this intricate process. Partial reprogramming, which rejuvenates cells without removing their specialized roles, holds considerable promise, and AI facilitates this research by balancing rejuvenation and essential cellular stability.

In tissue engineering and 3D bioprinting, AI precisely designs biologically accurate scaffolds mimicking the body's extracellular matrix. Through careful layering of cell-infused bioinks, AI systematically constructs viable tissues, using real-time monitoring to ensure optimal cell distribution, scaffold porosity, and biochemical gradients. Although simpler structures like cartilage, skin, and vascular grafts have been successfully bioprinted, creating fully functional organs remains an ambitious future goal.

A significant obstacle in engineered tissues is vascularization, crucial for tissue survival after transplantation. AI addresses this by predicting endothelial cell behaviors and guiding the formation of effective blood vessel networks. Deep learning models trained on natural vascular processes help create tissues capable of successful integration with the body's circulatory system, gradually moving tissue engineering closer to practical clinical use.

AI further addresses organ shortages through innovations like xenotransplantation—transplanting genetically modified animal organs into humans. AI evaluates immune responses to refine genetic modifications in donor animals, advancing this approach toward clinical feasibility. Additionally, AI supports the development of bioartificial organs, combining biological tissues and synthetic components for enhanced compatibility, function, and durability.

As regenerative medicine evolves, AI continues enabling personalized, data-driven interventions to restore aging tissues effectively. Through guiding biological repair and rejuvenation, AI presents compelling possibilities for extending healthy lifespans. Thoughtful integration, rigorous validation, and ethical oversight remain essential to ensure these innovations genuinely improve patient care and redefine clinical approaches to aging.

Intelligent Machines and Aging Bodies: AI and Robotics in the Longevity Revolution

Artificial intelligence (AI) and robotics are increasingly influencing aging by enhancing medical care, mobility, rehabilitation, and elder support. AI efficiently processes extensive datasets to predict health risks and tailor interventions, while robotics offers tangible physical assistance. Together, these technologies support older adults, promoting resilience, functionality, and autonomy to enhance longevity.

Robotic-assisted surgery clearly illustrates these advancements. Traditional surgical methods often involve large incisions, prolonged recoveries, and increased risks, particularly for aging patients. Systems like the da Vinci Surgical System increase precision through minimally invasive techniques, providing surgeons exceptional dexterity, stabilized movements, and magnified visualization. These improvements reduce surgical trauma, accelerating recovery and effectively extending healthspan.

In rehabilitation and mobility support, intelligent robotic exoskeletons dynamically analyze movement patterns, offering tailored assistance. Companies such as Ekso Bionics and ReWalk Robotics develop wearable devices that restore mobility, strengthen muscles, boost circulation, and mitigate risks of osteoporosis and deep vein thrombosis, thereby significantly improving health outcomes of people affected by these conditions.

AI further advances prosthetic technology, enabling bionic limbs to function as adaptive, intuitive extensions of the body. Unlike traditional prosthetics, AI-driven limbs utilize neural interfaces and machine learning to naturally respond to user intentions. Companies like BrainCo and Open Bionics design prosthetics that adapt seamlessly to user movements, improving control and dexterity. Innovations such as haptic feedback and proprioception, while promising, remain experimental and require further refinement.

AI and robotics are also evolving elder care through socially assistive robots and intelligent home automation. Robots such as Japan's Pepper and the PARO robotic seal provide emotional companionship, monitor vital signs, and assist with daily tasks, effectively reducing loneliness and caregiver strain. AI-enabled home systems support autonomous living through activity monitoring, fall detection, and automatic environmental adjustments, complementing human caregiving and raising important ethical considerations around privacy and autonomy.

Finally, as discussed in an earlier chapter, nanorobotics—microscopic robots operating at the cellular level—represent an exciting frontier in longevity science. AI-guided nanobots could soon deliver targeted treatments and cellular repairs, potentially enabling early disease detection and precise interventions for conditions like cancer and neurodegenerative diseases. While substantial technological challenges remain, ongoing research continues to push this groundbreaking field forward.

As AI and robotics mature, aging care moves from reactive treatments toward proactive strategies. By harnessing intelligent automation, advanced surgical techniques, enhanced mobility solutions, and targeted caregiving, these groundbreaking technologies rewrite the narrative of aging, fostering sustained independence and greater overall health.

Mind and Machine: How AI Supports Cognitive and Emotional Longevity

As lifespans extend further into our golden years, safeguarding cognitive health and emotional well-being becomes increasingly crucial. Medical breakthroughs have significantly lengthened life expectancy, yet maintaining mental clarity and emotional balance amidst age-related challenges remains vital. How can we sustain mental sharpness and emotional resilience as we age? Artificial intelligence (AI) provides compelling answers, offering innovative tools for early cognitive detection, tailored therapeutic support, adaptive cognitive training, and enhanced public health monitoring. By integrating AI-based insights into traditional medical and psychological practices, researchers are reenvisioning the possibilities for enduring mental vitality and emotional stability.

One remarkable contribution of AI is its ability to detect neurodegenerative diseases—such as Alzheimer's, Parkinson's, and vascular dementia—long before symptoms appear. Unlike traditional diagnostics, AI methods harness powerful machine learning algorithms trained on extensive neurological datasets. Functional MRI scans, PET scans, EEG readings, and subtle linguistic or handwriting changes collectively form a detailed picture of early cognitive decline. Even minor shifts in vocabulary or speech complexity, according to research by IBM Watson and similar institutions, can accurately forecast cognitive deterioration, greatly enhancing current diagnostic capabilities.

Beyond diagnostics, AI is modernizing mental health care by offering immediate, customized, and accessible therapeutic support. Virtual therapy platforms like Woebot and Wysa use advanced natural language processing (NLP) to facilitate structured conversations grounded in Cognitive Behavioral Therapy (CBT). Operating around the clock, these platforms bypass traditional barriers—such as cost, geography, or limited provider availability—extending meaningful support to underserved populations. While not replacements for human therapists, they complement existing mental health services, offering timely interventions, fostering emotional strength, and reducing the stigma associated with seeking help.

AI also revitalizes cognitive training through dynamic, adaptive techniques. Traditional repetitive exercises often lead to user disengagement; however, algorithm-based platforms such as Lumosity, CogniFit, and Elevate continually recalibrate tasks based on real-time performance. This adaptive approach promotes neuroplasticity, stimulating the brain's ability to form new neural connections and enhancing cognitive function. Ongoing studies aim to clarify precisely how adaptive cognitive training impacts mental agility and delays cognitive decline.

Neurofeedback technology benefits significantly from AI integration. EEG-based wearables, such as Muse and Emotiv, offer real-time brainwave monitoring, enabling users to develop customized meditation and mindfulness routines tailored to individual stress and focus levels. Continued research will further reveal the true extent to which these personalized interventions foster lasting cognitive health and emotional well-being.

Precision psychiatry represents another area dramatically transformed by AI. Rather than traditional trial-and-error prescribing methods, AI-enabled pharmacogenomics analyzes genetic profiles and neurotransmitter pathways to predict medication efficacy and side effects accurately. This precision approach can significantly optimize treatment outcomes, reducing adverse reactions and improving global mental healthcare quality. Further research and careful regulatory oversight will establish how precision psychiatry can become a standardized practice worldwide.

On a broader scale, AI influences public mental health monitoring by delivering timely, actionable insights into emerging mental health trends. Algorithms sift through social media data, search patterns, and wearable health metrics to detect signals of anxiety, depression, or elevated suicide risks. Public health organizations can allocate resources more effectively, implement targeted interventions, and enhance community mental health support. Nevertheless, ethical considerations regarding privacy, data security, and algorithmic fairness should remain at the forefront.

As AI integrates into diagnostics, therapy, cognitive enhancement, neurofeedback, and public health strategies, its potential to sustain mental longevity continues to expand. By proactively addressing the cognitive and emotional challenges associated with aging, AI-guided research promises a future characterized not only by longer lives but by enriched quality, enduring mental vitality, and sustained emotional well-being.

The Intelligent Future: AI, Aging, and the Promise of a New Era

Artificial intelligence (AI) is changing our perception of aging, transforming it from passive acceptance to active intervention through precise strategies designed to slow its progression and enhance quality of life. By integrating predictive analytics, regenerative medicine, cognitive enhancement, and molecular insights, AI-driven research enables preventive approaches that maintain vitality well before declines occur.

The growing role of AI in longevity science carries significant societal implications. Predictive modeling allows policymakers to anticipate medical resource needs, workforce changes, and economic adjustments due to demographic shifts. This foresight fosters sustainable healthcare systems, adaptive employment structures, and innovative retirement models. A future characterized by longer, healthier lives necessitates updating education, employment, and economic policies to support ongoing productivity and meaningful engagement.

While critical questions about aging remain unanswered, AI-enhanced research continues to illuminate previously unseen pathways—revealing intricate interactions, hidden synergies, and unexpected opportunities. Such insights not only hold promise for extending lifespan but also inspire innovative approaches that nurture personal growth, deepen self-understanding, and enrich the human experience at every stage of life.

CHAPTER 23

Partnering with Your Healthcare Provider: Building a Longevity Team

"The doctor of the future will give no medicine, but will interest his patients in the care of the human frame, in diet, and in the cause and prevention of disease."
—THOMAS EDISON

In previous chapters, we've explored the scientific, philosophical, and practical dimensions of longevity in substantial detail. Now, as we approach the conclusion of this book, the focus shifts deliberately—from detailed analysis to practical orientation. Chapter 23 introduces essential principles to help you build meaningful and effective relationships with your healthcare providers. Chapter 24 provides a structured yet flexible framework to transform your longevity ambitions into a clear, personalized plan. While these final chapters do not offer exhaustive instructions, they do provide strategic clarity and direction, empowering you to take your next steps toward greater longevity with confidence.

Modern medicine excels at managing acute illnesses, infections, and emergencies, significantly extending human lifespans. Yet chronic conditions remain a persistent challenge as people age. Conventional healthcare efficiently addresses immediate problems but frequently overlooks insidious biological changes linked to aging, typically focusing on symptom relief rather than addressing the underlying mechanisms driving functional decline and chronic disease. Routine checkups and preventive screenings, though crucial, often fall short in detecting early physiological signs of deterioration, allowing conditions such as cellular stress, mitochondrial impairment, chronic inflammation, hormonal disruptions, and metabolic imbalances to progress silently and become increasingly difficult to reverse.

Adding complexity, aging unfolds differently in each person. Even with identical diagnoses like elevated cholesterol or prediabetes, outcomes vary greatly due to genetics, metabolism, lifestyle, and hormonal status. Standard treatment guidelines, although helpful in general, cannot adequately account for this biological diversity.

Proactive by Design: Evolving Healthcare for Sustained Wellness

Longevity encompasses not just living longer, but maintaining physical strength, cognitive clarity, and emotional fulfillment deep into older age. To achieve these outcomes, healthcare must shift from a reactive to a proactive model—emphasizing early detection, ongoing monitoring, and tailored interventions.

Medical technology and diagnostics have advanced significantly, enabling earlier detection of health risks while the body's natural repair mechanisms remain robust. Just as reinforcing structural supports before damage occurs prevents a building's decline, prompt interventions can likewise avert deeper health deterioration. Longevity-oriented healthcare targets aging's core biological drivers, including cardiovascular, metabolic, and neurodegenerative diseases. Precision diagnostics combined with tailored lifestyle interventions enable healthcare professionals to create personalized wellness plans aligned with each person's unique biology. This shift enhances both physical and mental capacities, thereby improving quality of life and longevity.

A Multidisciplinary Approach

Optimizing lifespan and healthspan requires integrating conventional medical practices with advanced, longevity-focused interventions. Collaboration anchors this holistic model, as primary care physicians, longevity specialists, and allied health professionals coordinate to design individualized wellness strategies that adapt as health needs evolve.

Individual engagement is equally crucial. Equipped with clear education, accessible technologies, and personalized guidance, patients actively participate in their healthcare journey, ensuring longevity strategies remain sustainable and effective.

Architects of Longevity: The Role of Anti-Aging Specialists

Anti-aging and longevity specialists hold a pivotal role within preventive healthcare by identifying and addressing biological processes that accelerate aging before symptoms arise. Leveraging comprehensive assessments and advanced diagnostics, these specialists detect emerging risks early, creating timely intervention opportunities.

They translate detailed health data into personalized wellness plans incorporating nutritional strategies, targeted supplements, precision exercise programs, and evidence-based hormonal therapies. Care pathways evolve continually, reflecting new scientific insights and shifting health priorities. Importantly, anti-aging specialists coordinate with primary care providers and other medical professionals to recommend cohesive optimal aging practices.

Moreover, anti-aging specialists empower patients by providing practical methods for improving sleep, managing stress, enhancing movement, and promoting recovery. This holistic approach merges conventional medicine with advanced preventive strategies, guiding people toward sustained physical capability, cognitive resilience, and enriched quality of life.

Creating an Effective Healthcare Team

Building a healthcare team tailored specifically to your long-term wellness objectives demands thoughtful planning and flexibility. Begin by selecting a primary care physician who emphasizes preventive care, encourages shared decision-making, and genuinely values your perspective. If your current doctor is resistant to longevity-focused modalities or seems dismissive of your concerns, consider finding a clinician whose practice combines conventional medicine with forward-looking perspectives on aging and health optimization.

When evaluating longevity specialists, prioritize alignment with your goals. Do they actively stay current with advances in aging science? Are they committed to designing individualized protocols instead of relying on generic treatments? Directly inquire about their approaches to prevention, diagnostic precision, and collaboration with other providers.

It is valuable to emphasize that remote consultations via telemedicine, health coaching networks, and patient-driven research platforms can broaden access to specialized expertise regardless of geographic limitations. Facilitating regular communication among your providers is essential—though not always automatic. You might need to actively share medical records or encourage providers to collaborate directly. Hiring a health advocate or care coordinator can help streamline communication, particularly if or when managing complex or multi-specialist care.

Be mindful of logistical and financial considerations. Insurance coverage may exclude longevity-focused consultations, advanced diagnostics, or functional medicine services. If costs become a barrier, prioritize high-impact interventions or collaborate with providers offering tiered services.

View team-building as iterative: reassess periodically to align your team with evolving health needs, knowledge, and personal objectives.

A Foundation of Trust and Flexibility

Select healthcare providers who demonstrate curiosity, adaptability, and dedication to staying at the forefront of longevity science. Providers should offer clear, consistent communication, facilitating a responsive approach that evolves seamlessly with your changing health priorities. By thoughtfully curating a healthcare team grounded in mutual trust, interdisciplinary expertise, and rigorous, personalized protocols, you position yourself to fully harness your potential—achieving not only a longer life, but sustained adaptability in the face of change, dynamic engagement with the world around you, and a lifelong path of personal discovery.

CHAPTER 24

From Ambition to Clarity: Crafting Your Personal Longevity Strategy

"A goal without a plan is just a wish."
—Antoine de Saint-Exupéry

Two people might share the goal of living longer, healthier lives, yet their paths can differ dramatically. One proceeds deliberately, guided by thoughtful, adaptable, science-based goals, while the other experiments impulsively with diets, supplements, and routines, pursuing quick results without a clear vision. Although both have equal access to scientific knowledge, only the person who plans intentionally and consistently translates that knowledge into meaningful, lasting improvements.

A well-designed longevity plan provides more than just structure—it offers clarity and reassurance amid complexity. In an expanding landscape of scientifically validated therapies and experimental biohacks, having a clear, personalized roadmap helps filter distractions, highlights meaningful choices, and aligns daily routines with deeper biological principles. Without this intentional approach, we risk becoming reactive to health issues rather than proactively preventing them. Purposeful decisions, made consistently, yield lasting and meaningful benefits.

No single approach guarantees longevity, nor does a universal solution exist. Scientific evidence confirms that aging is highly modifiable, yet individual responses vary significantly due to genetics and personal biology. For instance, intermittent fasting may enhance cellular repair and metabolism in some people but trigger hormonal imbalances or heightened stress in others. Similarly, antioxidant supplements might reduce inflammation and boost vitality for certain people, yet paradoxically accelerate aging or impair physiological function in others. Even universally beneficial practices such as exercise require thoughtful personalization according to age, physical capability, and unique life circumstances.

Longevity emerges not from isolated habits but from mutually reinforcing practices. Strategies such as mindful nutrition, tailored exercise routines, and restorative sleep synergistically support overall well-being. A thoughtfully crafted health plan identifies and amplifies these connections, emphasizing sustainable results rather than temporary fixes.

This chapter connects theory to practical application, guiding you through purposeful, evidence-based actions that meaningfully shape your experience of aging. While growing older is an unavoidable reality, you have significant control over how the process unfolds. Customized lifestyle choices, targeted health interventions, and evolving medical technologies present genuine, achievable opportunities to extend both healthspan and lifespan.

The following sections provide practical tools for evaluating your current health status, prioritizing impactful choices, and integrating these insights into a flexible and evolving plan, responsive to scientific advances and personal changes.

Although aging itself cannot be avoided, the decisions you make—grounded in thoughtful, scientifically informed actions—actively define its trajectory. Deliberate habits unlock sustained mental sharpness, physical durability, and an enriched experience of life, placing these outcomes realistically within your grasp.

Know Thyself: Establishing Your Biological Basis for Lifelong Health

Every journey toward enhanced lifespan transforms broad aspirations into clear, personalized actions. The critical starting point is a comprehensive evaluation of your unique biological profile. Routine medical screenings, such as blood tests, lipid panels, fasting glucose measurements, and blood pressure readings, provide fundamental information about chronic disease risk and essential organ functions. However, thorough longevity assessments delve deeper, capturing vital physiological signals such as immune function, hormonal balance, genetic predispositions, and biomarkers of cellular aging.

Advanced diagnostics reveal early metabolic disturbances and hidden inflammation through specialized indicators like homocysteine and C-reactive protein (CRP). Cardiovascular health is evaluated by oxidative stress levels, fasting insulin, and triglyceride-to-HDL cholesterol ratios, while liver and kidney function tests measure organ resilience. Detailed hormone profiles—including testosterone, estrogen, thyroid function, and cortisol—help pinpoint imbalances impacting cognitive clarity, physical energy, and psychological stability.

For those interested in a deeper and more contemporary understanding of aging, assessing biological age can be remarkably insightful. Epigenetic testing explores DNA methylation patterns influenced by daily habits and environmental experiences, while telomere-length analysis provides valuable clues into cellular aging and regeneration. Evaluating mitochondrial function sheds light on how effectively your cells produce energy—a key to sustained vitality and resilience.

Practical physical measures, including grip strength, gait speed, muscle mass, bone density, and cardiovascular endurance (VO_2 max), offer concrete indicators of your overall fitness and functional health. Mental wellness evaluations—such as memory recall, reaction time, and cognitive processing speed—complement these physical assessments, painting a fuller picture of your neurological health. Finally, examining factors like sleep quality, emotional well-being, and stress resilience completes this integrative mosaic, empowering you to cultivate a nuanced, deeply personal understanding of your health journey.

Innovative tracking technologies—such as wearable devices including continuous glucose monitors, smartwatches, and health-tracking rings—further enhance your profile, supplying real-time data on heart-rate variability, glucose regulation, sleep patterns, and autonomic nervous system function.

Establishing this comprehensive and adaptive baseline allows for precise interpretation of your health data and the development of targeted, personalized protocols.

From Insight to Action: Interpreting Your Personal Health Profile

With your comprehensive biological benchmark established, the critical next step involves carefully interpreting this data. Like studying a detailed map before setting out on a journey, your biological, mental, and emotional assessments provide clarity about your current health status, helping to chart a purposeful path forward.

Begin by identifying significant patterns within your biomarkers. Pinpoint potential vulnerabilities, such as chronic inflammation, insulin resistance, or hormonal imbalances, and recognize strengths, such as cardiovascular fitness or muscular strength. Objectively evaluate how your lifestyle and genetic predispositions align or diverge from long-term health objectives, critically reviewing dietary practices, exercise habits, sleep quality, and stress-management routines. Genetic insights and family history should guide preventive decisions rather than determine outcomes.

Mental and emotional health dimensions also warrant close scrutiny. Identify neurological vulnerabilities or psychological stressors requiring proactive management. Acknowledge cognitive clarity and emotional resilience as significant assets.

At this analytical stage, emphasize achievable strategies instead of multiple simultaneous interventions. Clearly define outcomes—such as improved cardiovascular function, optimized metabolism, or enhanced neurological sharpness—matched precisely to your aspirations. Consider using structured goal-setting frameworks like SMART goals (*Specific*, clearly stating what is desired; *Measurable*, quantifying progress; *Achievable*, realistically attainable; *Relevant*, aligned with broader objectives; *Time-bound*, anchored to specific timelines). Applying such a systematic approach provides focus, enhances motivation, and significantly improves the likelihood of reaching meaningful, sustainable health outcomes.

From Aspirations to Achievement: Turning Health Goals into Tangible Results

How can priorities be translated into measurable outcomes? Effective planning involves establishing clear yet adaptable goals aligned with shifting health priorities and desired results. Clearly distinguish primary objectives—such as cardiovascular or neurological health—from secondary targets like better sleep quality or reduced stress. For example, metabolic objectives might aim to lower fasting glucose levels and enhance insulin sensitivity, whereas neurological goals could include regular cognitive assessments.

Establish a consistent method for tracking your progress—such as keeping a health journal, using a digital health dashboard, or consulting regularly with health professionals—to maintain alignment with evolving scientific developments and personal circumstances.

Blueprint for Lifelong Health: Building a Maintainable, Adaptive Lifestyle Plan

With clear goals established, focus next on sustainable implementation. Core lifestyle practices form a solid foundation. These include nutrition aimed at reducing inflammation and promoting cellular regeneration, balanced exercise integrating strength, cardiovascular, and mobility training, and consistent restorative sleep.

Targeted interventions amplify foundational habits. Periodic fasting stimulates autophagy and enhances cellular flexibility, high-intensity interval training (HIIT) boosts metabolic efficiency, and deliberate environmental stressors—such as heat or cold exposure—trigger beneficial physiological adaptations. Selective pharmacological and nutraceutical approaches, including senolytics and fasting-mimicking diets, can also be integrated based on validated research and individual biological profiles.

Your Wellness Team

Successfully implementing your personal health plan often requires collaboration with healthcare professionals. As detailed in Chapter 23: *Partnering with Your Healthcare Provider*, cultivating strong relationships with your primary care physician and wellness specialists ensures your approach remains safe, evidence-based, and adaptable to evolving health circumstances.

Balance Over Perfection: Navigating Common Challenges

One of the most frequent challenges on the journey to wellness is perfectionism, driven by unrealistic expectations that often lead to stress, frustration, and burnout. Science supports incremental, consistent progress over drastic, unsustainable measures—such as restrictive diets or excessively rigorous exercise routines—that rarely produce lasting results. Instead, aim to integrate manageable, evidence-based changes naturally into daily life, creating routines that feel intuitive rather than burdensome.

Regular monitoring of health markers can provide valuable insights, but science also cautions against the tension and anxiety resulting from excessive self-tracking—trust how you feel, prioritize balance, and emphasize progress over perfection. Additionally, recognize emotional and psychological well-being as fundamental to longevity. Cultivate meaningful social connections, nurture emotional flexibility, and engage in activities aligned with your personal values and sense of fulfillment. In essence, a balanced strategy blending scientific accuracy with self-compassion supports sustained health, lasting resilience, and greater overall satisfaction.

The Feedback Loop: Monitoring and Refining Your Health Strategy

An effective wellness strategy must evolve continuously, adapting in response to new scientific insights and personal developments. After establishing your initial baseline and structured goals, ongoing refinement ensures that your plan remains effective and relevant.

Scheduled periodic evaluations—semi-annually, annually, or after significant life events—provide meaningful data-driven insights into changes in biomarkers, physical fitness, and neurological performance. Wearable technologies and routine tracking enhance this feedback loop by capturing ongoing trends rather than isolated data points.

Integrating objective measurements with professional consultation and personal reflection ensures your health trajectory remains dynamic, scientifically valid, and responsive to evolving health conditions and life circumstances. This iterative monitoring and adaptation process helps maintain alignment with your long-term goals, enhancing the sustainability and effectiveness of your longevity program.

> *"What gets measured gets done. What gets measured and fed back gets done well. What gets rewarded gets repeated."*
> —JOHN E. JONES III

Bringing It All Together: Creating a Sustainable Longevity Plan

Having assessed your biology, interpreted your health profile, defined your priorities, and selected appropriate interventions, the next essential step is to construct a clear, practical blueprint for transforming insights into lasting habits. This framework must authentically align with your individual lifestyle, aspirations, and personal circumstances. Its power lies in its practicality, moving beyond theoretical ideas by explicitly outlining flexible routines that can be easily integrated into daily life.

A successful longevity strategy is expressed not just through intangible outcomes such as increased energy or enhanced mental clarity, but through the consistent rhythm of everyday life—aligned seamlessly with enduring personal values like intellectual curiosity, physical autonomy, emotional equilibrium, and meaningful contributions to family and community. Guided by this expansive vision, your primary objective shifts toward nurturing consistency: creating a structured yet flexible framework that readily adapts to life's inevitable changes.

Begin by defining a personal routine customized to your responsibilities and commitments. Establish clear checkpoints—daily reflections, weekly reviews, and quarterly assessments—to ensure accountability, track progress, and facilitate timely adjustments. Clearly document your longevity plan in writing. This evolving document, flexible yet purposeful, grows richer through ongoing experience and new discoveries, serving as a trusted reference amid life's continuous evolution.

Thoughtful and consistent planning becomes an essential discipline—an embodiment of personal agency and foresight. This organized yet flexible method lays a robust foundation for deeper explorations of mindful living, shifting the emphasis from simply extending life toward enhancing its inherent quality and significance.

Aging with Intention: Designing a Purpose-Driven Life

At the intersection of art, science, and practical strategy lies conscious living—the culmination and true mastery of your wellness journey. While knowledge and scientific innovation provide essential tools, genuine fulfillment arises when mindful health practices become seamlessly integrated into daily life. Nourishing your body thoughtfully, prioritizing physical activity, ensuring restful sleep, and cultivating emotional resilience no longer remain tasks to do but become second nature, enriching the quality of everyday experiences.

This may include refining your nutritional habits, enhancing sleep hygiene, proactively engaging with health assessments, or consulting experts in the field. Over time, successful wellness planning accommodates personal circumstances and integrates new scientific discoveries, balancing innovative enthusiasm with consistent adherence to foundational health principles.

The core of conscious living transcends lifespan extension alone, elevating your life's quality and significance by blending multiple dimensions of wellness into a cohesive, meaningful lifestyle. As foundational habits solidify, you can explore advanced strategies—pharmaceutical innovations offering increased vitality or powerful non-pharmacological practices enhancing daily engagement and well-being.

Looking ahead, breakthroughs in regenerative medicine, gene therapy, emerging technologies, and artificial intelligence will continually redefine aging possibilities. Collaborating actively with your healthcare providers ensures that these advances meaningfully enhance your personalized wellness strategy. Mindful living transforms longevity from just accumulation of years into a meaningful journey—guided by curiosity, enriched by rewarding experiences, and open to ongoing exploration of aging's potential.

Live deliberately, live consciously, live with meaning, live with purpose...

> *"Life is never made unbearable by circumstances, but only by lack of meaning and purpose"*
> —Victor Frankl

Postscript

The Age of Possibility: A Final Reflection

Aging was once seen as an unstoppable force—an inevitable part of the human condition. It was something to endure, resist, or, at best, postpone. Today, our understanding has evolved dramatically. Aging is no longer perceived as a singular event but as a dynamic, ongoing process, influenced by biology, time, and deliberate human choices.

Historically, longevity depended primarily on genetics, luck, and the limitations of medical understanding. We now stand at a remarkable threshold where knowledge translates directly into empowerment. The body does not merely wear out; rather, it follows biological programs we have begun to understand—programs we can optimize, enhance, or perhaps even rewrite. Cellular repair can be strengthened, cognitive decline mitigated, and physical strength, once thought the exclusive province of youth, maintained far longer than previously imagined.

Longevity is more than scientific advancement; it is a philosophy, a conscious approach to life itself. A longer life is meaningful only if filled with purpose, energy, and active engagement. The true measure of longevity lies not in accumulated years but in how richly those years are experienced—the ideas pursued, relationships nurtured, and moments created.

Throughout this book, strategies have been provided to extend healthspan, optimize physical and cognitive function, and challenge conventional narratives of aging. But reading about longevity is not the same as living it. Knowledge alone does not transform your journey; it must become action.

A longevity plan is sustained by daily habits and a clear sense of intention integrated into everyday decisions.

Science continually refines our understanding, yet certain truths remain timeless. No drug, genetic intervention, or scientific breakthrough surpasses the fundamental elements of a meaningful life: curiosity, purpose, and genuine human connection. Longevity is neither a number nor a denial of mortality—it is an opportunity to awaken each day with strength, clarity, and a deep awareness that life still holds much to offer.

Perhaps the most important realization is that aging is not something that simply happens to us. We actively participate in the process. Every meal, every movement, each restful night, and every meaningful conversation matters. In the quiet, ordinary moments of daily life, we shape our future.

As our power over personal aging grows, we must acknowledge broader implications. Longevity has become more than an individual aspiration—it is now a societal transformation. When we reject aging as predetermined decline and embrace it as an adventure, we reimagine our understanding of work, relationships, community, and purpose. As scientific progress accelerates, an essential question emerges: What will we choose to do with the additional time we gain?

This question remains unanswered, and the future of aging is ours to write. The path ahead is expansive, uncharted, and full of possibility. Live boldly. Age vibrantly. Embrace each moment deliberately—and trust that your most meaningful moments are yet to come.

Drs. Ioulia and Don Howard

> *"What we call the beginning is often the end. And*
> *to make an end is to make a beginning."*
> —T. S. Eliot

References

About These References
The references included in this section provide the scientific foundation for the strategies, research, and concepts explored throughout this book. Covering historical and philosophical perspectives on aging as well as emerging advancements in longevity science, these sources support our discussions on physical activity, nutrition, supplements, fasting, sleep, stress management, emotional well-being, sex, hormonal health, pharmacological interventions, biohacking, regenerative medicine, gene therapy, artificial intelligence, and personalized longevity planning.

To enhance usability, references are organized by subject rather than in a single alphabetical list, enabling readers to efficiently locate information relevant to specific topics of interest. Within each category, references are arranged alphabetically by the first author's last name and formatted according to APA (7th edition) guidelines. Digital object identifiers (DOIs) or URLs have been provided wherever available, facilitating direct access to original research articles, authoritative reports, and key texts.

Although the references included here comprehensively represent key studies and authoritative sources in longevity science, it's essential to recognize that this field remains expansive, intricate, and continually evolving. Our aim in this book has been to distill that complexity into clear, engaging, and practically relevant content—balancing thoroughness with readability, and emphasizing broad insights rather than exhaustive technical detail. Some nuances have been deliberately streamlined to enhance accessibility, and ongoing debates or finer details may be best explored through specialized scientific literature. Thus, the scientific depth provided is intentionally matched to the interests and needs of an intelligent, scientifically curious reader rather than the exhaustive standards of specialists. Readers seeking further exploration are encouraged to regularly consult peer-reviewed journals, publications from academic institutions, expert-reviewed literature, and other reputable resources. We invite active participation in this exciting field—encouraging curiosity, critical inquiry, and continual discovery—because the science of longevity, much like life itself, is dynamic and ever-unfolding.

History of Aging

Achenbaum, W. A. (2013). A historical perspective in aging and gerontology. In D. Dannefer & C. Phillipson (Eds.), The SAGE handbook of social gerontology (pp. 3–13). SAGE Publications. https://doi.org/10.4135/9781446200933.n2

Center for Healthy Aging. (2022, February 21). History of aging research. Colorado State University. https://www.research.colostate.edu/healthyagingcenter/2022/02/21/history-of-aging-research/

Chappel, J. (2024). Golden years: How Americans invented and reinvented old age. Atlantic Books. https://www.theatlantic.com/magazine/archive/2025/01/james-chappel-golden-years-andrew-j-scott-longevity-imperative/680762/

Dowling, M., Kenney, C., & Carney, M. T. (2024). The aging revolution: The history of geriatric health care and what really matters to older adults. Northwell Health Press. https://www.johnahartford.org/dissemination-center/view/the-aging-revolution-the-history-of-geriatric-health-care-and-what-really-matters-to-older-adults-northwell-health

Haber, C. (2011). A cultural and economic history of old age in America. Mayo Clinic Proceedings, 86(9), 848–850. https://doi.org/10.4065/mcp.2011.0265

Katz, S. (2018). Aging through the lens of historical time, space, and place. The Gerontologist, 58(4), 795–802. https://doi.org/10.1093/geront/gnx195

University of Cambridge. (2010, May 24). A brief history of ageing. University of Cambridge News. https://www.cam.ac.uk/research/news/a-brief-history-of-ageing

Philosophy and Aging

Aristotle. (2019). Nicomachean ethics. Cambridge University Press.

Frankl, V. E. (2006). Man's search for meaning. Beacon Press.

Marcus Aurelius. (2002). Meditations (G. Hays, Trans.). Modern Library.

Nietzsche, F. (1992). Ecce homo. Penguin Classics.

Seneca. (2004). On the shortness of life. Penguin Classics.

Buettner, D. (2012). The Blue Zones: Lessons for living longer from the people who've lived the longest. National Geographic.

Davidson, R. J., & McEwen, B. S. (2012). Social influences on neuroplasticity: Stress and interventions to promote well-being. Nature Neuroscience, 15(5), 689–695. https://doi.org/10.1038/nn.3093

Ryff, C. D., & Singer, B. H. (1998). The contours of positive human health. Psychological Inquiry, 9(1), 1–28. https://doi.org/10.1207/s15327965pli0901_1

Waldinger, R., & Schulz, M. (2023). The good life: Lessons from the world's longest scientific study of happiness. Simon & Schuster.

Weil, A. (2005). Healthy aging: A lifelong guide to your well-being. Knopf.

García, H., & Miralles, F. (2017). Ikigai: The Japanese secret to a long and happy life. Penguin Books.

Haidt, J. (2006). The happiness hypothesis: Finding modern truth in ancient wisdom. Basic Books.

Purpose and Longevity

Epel, E. S., et al. (2009). Meditation practice is associated with longer telomeres in women. Annals of the New York Academy of Sciences, 1172, 34–53. https://doi.org/10.1196/annals.1393.001

Hill, P. L., & Turiano, N. A. (2014). Purpose in life as a predictor of mortality across adulthood. Psychological Science, 25(7), 1482–1486. https://doi.org/10.1177/0956797614531799

Holt-Lunstad, J., Smith, T. B., & Layton, J. B. (2010). Social relationships and mortality risk: A meta-analytic review. PLoS Medicine, 7(7), e1000316. https://doi.org/10.1371/journal.pmed.1000316

Sapolsky, R. M. (2004). Why zebras don't get ulcers. Holt Paperbacks.

Theories of Aging

Biological Theories of Aging

Aquino, T., & Leuzzi, L. (2025). Finite-size effects in aging can be interpreted as sub-aging. *arXiv.* https://arxiv.org/abs/2501.04843

Gems, D., & de Magalhães, J. P. (2021). The hoverfly and the wasp: A critique of the hallmarks of aging as a paradigm. *Ageing Research Reviews, 70,* Article 101407. https://doi.org/10.1016/j.arr.2021.101407

Kennedy, B. K., Berger, S. L., Brunet, A., Campisi, J., Cuervo, A. M., Epel, E. S., Franceschi, C., Lithgow, G. J., Morimoto, R. I., Pessin, J. E., Rando, T. A., Richardson, A., Schadt, E. E., Wyss-Coray, T., & Sierra, F. (2014). Geroscience: Linking aging to chronic disease. *Cell, 159*(4), 709–713. https://doi.org/10.1016/j.cell.2014.10.039

Lemaître, J. F., Ronget, V., & Gaillard, J. M. (2024). The evolution of ageing: Classic theories and emerging ideas. *Biogerontology, 25*(1), 1–15. https://doi.org/10.1007/s10522-024-10143-5

López-Otín, C., Blasco, M. A., Partridge, L., Serrano, M., & Kroemer, G. (2013). The hallmarks of aging. *Cell, 153*(6), 1194–1217. https://doi.org/10.1016/j.cell.2013.05.039

López-Otín, C., Blasco, M. A., Partridge, L., Serrano, M., & Kroemer, G. (2023). Hallmarks of aging: An expanding universe. *Cell, 186*(2), 243–278. https://doi.org/10.1016/j.cell.2022.12.038

Maklakov, A. A., & Regan, J. C. (2025). Consolidating multiple evolutionary theories of ageing suggests a need for new approaches to study genetic contributions to ageing decline. *Ageing Research Reviews.* Advance online publication. https://doi.org/10.1016/j.arr.2024.102201

Medawar, P. B. (1952). *An unsolved problem of biology.* H. K. Lewis.

Pridham, G., & Rutenberg, A. D. (2023). Dynamical network stability analysis of multiple biological ages provides a framework for understanding the aging process. *arXiv.* https://arxiv.org/abs/2309.10005

Qin, H. (2024). The emergent aging model: Aging as an emergent property of biological systems. *arXiv.* https://arxiv.org/abs/2407.05226

Tapias, D., Marteau, C., Aguirre-López, F., & Sollich, P. (2024). Bringing together two paradigms of non-equilibrium: Driven dynamics of aging systems. *arXiv.* https://arxiv.org/abs/2402.03516

The hallmarks of aging as a conceptual framework for health and disease. (2024). *Frontiers in Aging.* https://doi.org/10.3389/fragi.2024.1334261

Theories of aging: Advancing understanding in 2024. (2024). *Longevity.Technology.* https://longevity.technology/news/theories-of-aging-advancing-understanding-in-2024/

Viña, J., Borrás, C., & Miquel, J. (2007). Theories of ageing. *IUBMB Life, 59*(4–5), 249–254. https://doi.org/10.1080/15216540701226011

Wang, Y., & Zhu, L. (2025). Molecule-dynamic-based aging clock and aging roadmap forecast with Sundial. *arXiv.* https://arxiv.org/abs/2501.02176

Wang, Z., et al. (2024). Pro-aging metabolic reprogramming: A unified theory of aging. *Engineering.* Advance online publication. https://doi.org/10.1016/j.eng.2024.09.010

The Epigenetic Clock as a Measure of Biological Aging

Brigham and Women's Hospital. (2024, February 14). New epigenetic clocks reinvent how we measure age. ScienceDaily. Retrieved from https://www.sciencedaily.com/releases/2024/02/240214203341.htm

CheekAge. (2024). A next-generation epigenetic buccal clock predictive of mortality in human blood. Frontiers in Aging. https://doi.org/10.3389/fnagi.2024.01023

Garma, L., & Quintela-Fandino, M. (2024). Applicability of epigenetic age models to next-generation methylation arrays. Genome Medicine, 16(1), Article 116. https://doi.org/10.1186/s13073-024-0116-0

Leroy, A., Teh, A. L., Dondelinger, F., Alvarez, M. A., & Wang, D. (2023). Longitudinal prediction of DNA methylation to forecast epigenetic outcomes. arXiv. https://doi.org/10.48550/arXiv.2312.13302

Voisin, S., Harvey, N. R., Haupt, L. M., Griffiths, L. R., Ashton, K. J., & Coffey, V. G. (2023). Influence of physical activity on the epigenetic clock: Evidence from a monozygotic twin study. Clinical Epigenetics, 15, Article 56. https://doi.org/10.1186/s13148-023-01756-4

Psychological Theories of Aging

Min, J., Yoo, H. J., Nashiro, K., & Mather, M. (2024). Modulating heart rate oscillation affects plasma amyloid beta and tau levels in younger and older adults. *Scientific Reports, 13*, 12345. https://doi.org/10.1038/s41598-023-39453-1

Nashiro, K., Yoo, H. J., Min, J., & Mather, M. (2024). Increasing coordination and responsivity of emotion-related brain regions with a heart rate variability biofeedback randomized trial. *Cognitive, Affective, & Behavioral Neuroscience.* https://doi.org/10.3758/s13415-023-01100-7

Shenkman, G., Ifrah, K., & Shmotkin, D. (2023). The contribution of couplehood and parenthood to the hedonic and eudaimonic well-being of older gay men. *Journal of Happiness Studies, 24*, 1234–1250. https://doi.org/10.1007/s10902-022-00567-8

Stine-Morrow, E. A. L., West, R., Cheng, S., Abrams, L., Gerstorf, D., Hooker, K., Kunzmann, U., & Lustig, C. (2024). Advancing theory-driven research in the psychological science of adult development and aging. *Psychology and Aging, 39*(8). https://doi.org/10.1037/pag0000865

Sociological Theories of Aging

Katz, S. (2024). Sociology and gerontology: New perspectives and vital issues. *Innovation in Aging, 8*(Supplement_1), 601. https://doi.org/10.1093/geroni/igy023.601

Katz, S., & Marshall, B. L. (2024). New materialist insights in the sociology of aging: Rethinking agency and context. *Innovation in Aging, 8*(Supplement_1), 602. https://doi.org/10.1093/geroni/igy023.602

Sharma, M., & Sharma, S. (2023). Sociological theories of ageing and their influence on the quality of life of older adults. *Research and Reviews: Journal of Geriatric Nursing and Health Sciences, 9*(3), 17–22. https://matjournals.net/nursing/index.php/RRJGNHS/article/view/17

Shmotkin, D. (2023). Psychosocial and biological pathways to aging. *Zeitschrift für Gerontologie und Geriatrie, 56*(5), 482–489. https://doi.org/10.1007/s00391-024-02324-1

Exercise

Ahern, S., Sharma, R., & Mathes, D. (2025). Importance of exercise for career longevity, injury prevention, and mental health among plastic surgeons. Plastic and Reconstructive Surgery—Global Open, 13(1), e5256. https://doi.org/10.1097/GOX.0000000000005256

Andersen, K., Pedersen, B. K., Kujala, U. M., & Singh, M. A. F. (2025). Global exercise recommendations for healthy ageing: A multifaceted approach for older adults. Age and Ageing, 54(1), Article afad001. https://doi.org/10.1093/ageing/afad001

Booth, F. W., Roberts, C. K., & Laye, M. J. (2012). Lack of exercise is a major cause of chronic diseases. Comprehensive Physiology, 2(2), 1143–1211. https://doi.org/10.1002/cphy.c110025

Conroy, G. (2024, May 1). Why is exercise good for you? Scientists are finding answers in our cells. Nature News. Retrieved from https://www.nature.com/articles/example-url

D'Onofrio, G., Kirschner, J., Prather, H., Goldman, D., & Rozanski, A. (2023). Musculoskeletal exercise: Its role in promoting health and longevity. Progress in Cardiovascular Diseases, 77, 25–36. https://doi.org/10.1016/j.pcad.2023.02.006

Falshaw, N., Sagner, M., & Siow, R. C. (2024). The Longevity Med Summit: Insights on healthspan from cell to society. Frontiers in Aging, 5, Article 1417455. https://doi.org/10.3389/fragi.2024.1417455

Garber, C. E., Blissmer, B., Deschenes, M. R., et al. (2011). American College of Sports Medicine position stand. Quantity and quality of exercise for developing and maintaining cardiorespiratory, musculoskeletal, and neuromotor fitness in apparently healthy adults: Guidance for prescribing exercise. Medicine and Science in Sports and Exercise, 43(7), 1334–1359. https://doi.org/10.1249/MSS.0b013e318213fefb

Guan, Y., & Yan, Z. (2022). Molecular mechanisms of exercise and healthspan. Cells, 11(5), Article 872. https://doi.org/10.3390/cells11050872

Hamilton, K. L., & Selman, C. (2023). Can exercise prevent the age-related decline in adaptive homeostasis? Evidence across organisms and tissues. The Journal of Physiology. https://doi.org/10.1113/JP284583

Harvard Health Publishing. (2023). Adding weight lifting to workouts may boost longevity. Harvard Health. Retrieved from https://www.health.harvard.edu/heart-health/adding-weight-lifting-to-workouts-may-boost-longevity

Harvard Health Publishing. (2023). Strength training might lengthen life. Harvard Health. Retrieved from https://www.health.harvard.edu/staying-healthy/strength-training-might-lengthen-life

Harvard T.H. Chan School of Public Health. (2023). Exercising more than recommended could lengthen life, study suggests. Harvard T.H. Chan School of Public Health News. Retrieved from https://www.hsph.harvard.edu/news/hsph-in-the-news/exercising-more-than-recommended-could-lengthen-life-study-suggests/

Khan, M., Al Saud, H., Sierra, F., Perez, V., Greene, W., Al Asiry, S., Pathai, S., & Torres, M. (2024). Global Healthspan Summit 2023: Closing the gap between healthspan and lifespan. Nature Aging, 4(4), 445–448. https://doi.org/10.1038/s43587-024-00593-4

Lee, D. H., Rezende, L. F. M., Joh, H.-K., Keum, N., Ferrari, G., Rey-Lopez, J. P., Rimm, E. B., Tabung, F. K., & Giovannucci, E. L. (2022). Long-term leisure-time physical activity intensity and all-cause and cause-specific mortality: A prospective cohort of US adults. Circulation, 146(7). https://doi.org/10.1161/CIRCULATIONAHA.121.058162

McKee, A., Ortega, F. B., & Lavie, C. J. (2021). Exercise and lifespan: A genomic and epigenomic perspective. Progress in Cardiovascular Diseases, 64, 65–72. https://doi.org/10.1016/j.pcad.2020.12.002

Powell, K. E., King, A. C., Buchner, D. M., et al. (2019). The scientific foundation for the physical activity guidelines for Americans, 2nd edition. Journal of Physical Activity and Health, 16(1), 1–11. https://doi.org/10.1123/jpah.2018-0618

Ruegsegger, G. N., & Booth, F. W. (2018). Health benefits of exercise. Cold Spring Harbor Perspectives in Medicine, 8(7), Article a029694. https://doi.org/10.1101/cshperspect.a029694

Seals, D. R., Justice, J. N., & LaRocca, T. J. (2016). Physiological geroscience: Targeting function to increase healthspan and lifespan. The Journal of Physiology, 594(8), 2001–2024. https://doi.org/10.1113/JP270538

Swainson, M. G., Biddle, S. J. H., & Stamatakis, E. (2025). Physical activity intensity versus volume: Which matters more for reducing mortality risk? European Journal of Preventive Cardiology, 32(1), 10–11. https://doi.org/10.1093/eurjpc/zvad121

Vieira, R. F. L., Junqueira, R. L., Gaspar, R. C., Munoz, V. R., & Pauli, J. R. (2023). Exercise activates AMPK signaling: Impact on glucose uptake in the skeletal muscle in aging. Rehabilitation Journal. Retrieved from https://

www.rehabiljournal.com/articles/exercise-activates-ampk-signaling-impact-on-glucose-uptake-in-the-skeletal-muscle-in-aging.html

Warburton, D. E., & Bredin, S. S. (2017). Health benefits of physical activity: A systematic review of current systematic reviews. Current Opinion in Cardiology, 32(5), 541–556. https://doi.org/10.1097/HCO.0000000000000437

Additional News & Industry Sources (Non-peer-reviewed but relevant to understanding exercise and longevity.)

American Council on Exercise. (2023). Exercise and longevity: Empowering and motivating clients. *ACE Fitness*. https://www.acefitness.org/resources/pros/expert-articles/8752/exercise-and-longevity-empowering-and-motivating-clients/

American Council on Exercise. (2023). Longevity and exercise: Understanding lifespan vs. healthspan. *ACE Fitness*. https://www.acefitness.org/resources/pros/expert-articles/8730/the-longevity-buzzword-understanding-aging-lifespan-healthspan-and-the-role-of-exercise/

American Medical Association. (2023). Massive study uncovers how much exercise is needed to live longer. *American Medical Association News*. https://www.ama-assn.org/delivering-care/public-health/massive-study-uncovers-how-much-exercise-needed-live-longer

GQ. (2023). What's the best workout for longevity? *GQ Magazine*. https://www.gq.com/story/best-workout-for-longevity

Legendary Strength. (2023). Surprising longevity insights from a new fitness study. *Legendary Strength Blog*. https://legendarystrength.com/surprising-longevity-insights-from-a-new-fitness-study/

OnePeloton. (2023). Exercise for longevity: Workout routines for a lengthy life. *Peloton Blog*. https://www.onepeloton.com/blog/exercise-for-longevity/

Nutrition and Diet

Bajerska, J., Chmurzynska, A., Muzsik, A., Krzyzanowska, P., Madry, E., Malinowska, A. M., & Walkowiak, J. (2018). Weight loss and metabolic health effects from energy-restricted Mediterranean and Central-European diets in postmenopausal women: A randomized controlled trial. *Scientific Reports*, 8, Article 11170. https://doi.org/10.1038/s41598-018-29495-3

Cabo, R. de, & Mattson, M. P. (2019). Effects of intermittent fasting on health, aging, and disease. New England Journal of Medicine, 381(26), 2541–2551. https://doi.org/10.1056/NEJMra1905136

Dong, L., Teh, D. B. L., Kennedy, B. K., et al. (2023). Unraveling female reproductive senescence to enhance healthy longevity. Cell Research, 33(1), 11–29. https://doi.org/10.1038/s41422-022-00718-7

Estruch, R., Ros, E., Salas-Salvadó, J., Covas, M. I., Corella, D., Arós, F., & Martínez-González, M. A. (2023). Primary prevention of cardiovascular disease with a Mediterranean diet supplemented with extra-virgin olive oil or nuts. The New England Journal of Medicine, 390(3), 390–401. https://doi.org/10.1056/NEJMoa1800389

Estruch, R., Ros, E., Salas-Salvadó, J., et al. (2018). Primary prevention of cardiovascular disease with a Mediterranean diet supplemented with extra-virgin olive oil or nuts. New England Journal of Medicine, 378(25), e34.

Fontana, L., & Partridge, L. (2023). Promoting health and longevity through diet: From model organisms to humans. Cell, 184(3), 1–17. https://doi.org/10.1016/j.cell.2023.03.002

Fraser, G. E., & Shavlik, D. J. (2001). Ten years of life: Is it a matter of choice? Archives of Internal Medicine, 161(13), 1645–1652. https://doi.org/10.1001/archinte.161.13.1645

Greenhill, C. (2024). The complex effects of dietary restriction on longevity and health. Nature Reviews Endocrinology, 20(10), 697. https://doi.org/10.1038/s41574-024-01051-2

Hu, F. B. (2023). Diet strategies for promoting healthy aging and longevity: An epidemiological perspective. Journal of Internal Medicine. https://doi.org/10.1111/joim.13728

Hu, F. B., et al. (2025). Healthy eating in midlife linked to overall healthy aging. Nature Medicine. https://doi.org/10.1038/s41591-025-01234-5

Jacquier, E. F., Kassis, A., Marcu, D., Contractor, N., Hong, J., Hu, C., Kuehn, M., Lenderink, C., & Rajgopal, A. (2024). Phytonutrients in the promotion of healthspan: A new perspective. Frontiers in Nutrition, 11. https://doi.org/10.3389/fnut.2024.1409339

Levine, M. E., Suarez, J. A., Brandhorst, S., Balasubramanian, P., Cheng, C. W., Madia, F., & Longo, V. D. (2014). Low protein intake is associated with a major reduction in IGF-1, cancer, and overall mortality in the 65 and younger but not older population. Cell Metabolism, 19(3), 407–417. https://doi.org/10.1016/j.cmet.2014.02.006

Longo, V. D., & Anderson, R. M. (2023). Nutrition, longevity and disease: From molecular mechanisms to interventions. Cell, 185(9), 145–156. https://doi.org/10.1016/j.cell.2023.09.022

MacArthur, M. R., & Mitchell, S. J. (2023). Sex differences in healthspan and lifespan responses to geroprotective dietary interventions in preclinical models. Current Opinion in Physiology, 33, 100651. https://doi.org/10.1016/j.cophys.2023.100651

Mattison, J. A., Colman, R. J., Beasley, T. M., Allison, D. B., & Anderson, R. M. (2024). Caloric restriction improves health and survival of rhesus monkeys. Nature Communications, 11(1), 1400–1410. https://doi.org/10.1038/s41467-024-01122-z

Mishra, A., Giuliani, G., & Longo, V. D. (2024). Nutrition and dietary restrictions in cancer prevention. Biochimica et Biophysica Acta (BBA) - Reviews on Cancer, 1879(1), 189063. https://doi.org/10.1016/j.bbcan.2023.189063

Morris, M. C., Tangney, C. C., Wang, Y., Sacks, F. M., Barnes, L. L., Bennett, D. A., & Aggarwal, N. T. (2015). MIND diet associated with reduced incidence of Alzheimer's disease. *Alzheimer's & Dementia: The Journal of the Alzheimer's Association*, 11(9), 1007–1014. https://doi.org/10.1016/j.jalz.2014.11.009

Morze, J., Danielewicz, A., Przybyłowicz, K., Zeng, H., Hoffmann, G., & Schwingshackl, L. (2021). An updated systematic review and meta-analysis on adherence to Mediterranean diet and risk of cancer. *European Journal of Nutrition*, 60(3), 1561–1586. https://doi.org/10.1007/s00394-020-02346-6

Park, S.-H., Lee, D.-H., Lee, D.-H., & Jung, C. H. (2024). Scientific evidence of foods that improve the lifespan and healthspan of different organisms. Nutrition Research Reviews, 37(1), 169–178. https://doi.org/10.1017/S0954422423000136

Schwingshackl, L., & Hoffmann, G. (2014). Adherence to Mediterranean diet and risk of cancer: An updated systematic review and meta-analysis of observational studies. *International Journal of Cancer*, 135(8), 1884–1897. https://doi.org/10.1002/ijc.28824

Wilhelmi de Toledo, F., Grundler, F., Sirtori, C. R., & Ruscica, M. (2024). Intermittent fasting: From molecular effects to clinical implications in human health. Trends in Endocrinology & Metabolism, 34(1), 21–33. https://doi.org/10.1016/j.tem.2024.01.003

Willcox, D. C., et al. (2025). Demographic, phenotypic, and genetic characteristics of centenarians in Okinawa and Japan: Part 1—Centenarians in Okinawa. Journal of Gerontology: Medical Sciences. https://doi.org/10.1093/gerona/glab123

Zhang, Y., et al. (2025). A dietary swap that could lengthen your life? The American Journal of Clinical Nutrition. https://doi.org/10.1093/ajcn/nqaa123

Alcohol and Aging

Centers for Disease Control and Prevention. (n.d.). About alcohol use and your health. Retrieved December 16, 2024, from https://www.cdc.gov/alcohol/about-alcohol-use/index.html

Centers for Disease Control and Prevention. (n.d.). Moderate alcohol use. Retrieved December 16, 2024, from https://www.cdc.gov/alcohol/about-alcohol-use/moderate-alcohol-use.html

National Institute on Alcohol Abuse and Alcoholism. (n.d.). What are U.S. guidelines for drinking? Retrieved December 16, 2024, from https://rethinkingdrinking.niaaa.nih.gov/how-much-too-much/what-are-us-guidelines-drinking

U.S. News & World Report. (2024, August 13). Even light drinking harms health of older adults, study finds. Retrieved from https://www.usnews.com/news/health-news/articles/2024-08-13/even-light-drinking-harms-health-of-older-adults-study

World Health Organization. (2023). No level of alcohol consumption is safe for our health. Retrieved December 16, 2024, from https://www.who.int/europe/news-room/04-01-2023-no-level-of-alcohol-consumption-is-safe-for-our-health

World Health Organization. (2024). Over 3 million annual deaths due to alcohol and drug use. Retrieved December 16, 2024, from https://www.who.int/news/item/25-06-2024-over-3-million-annual-deaths-due-to-alcohol-and-drug-use-majority-among-men

Zheng, L., Liao, W., Luo, S., Li, B., Liu, D., Yun, Q., Zhao, Z., Zhao, J., Rong, J., Gong, Z., Sha, F., & Tang, J. (2024). Association between alcohol consumption and incidence of dementia in current drinkers: Linear and non-linear Mendelian randomization analysis. EClinicalMedicine, 76, 102810. https://doi.org/10.1016/j.eclinm.2024.102810

Supplements and Functional Foods: Peer-Reviewed Research and Scientific Studies

Kumar, R., Ng, D., & Wagner, K. H. (2022). GlyNAC supplementation improves glutathione deficiency, oxidative stress, mitochondrial dysfunction, and extends lifespan in aged mice. Free Radical Biology and Medicine, 174, 209–221. https://doi.org/10.1016/j.freeradbiomed.2021.11.013

Macpherson, H., Peters, R., & Leach, C. (2013). Multivitamins and mortality: A systematic review and meta-analysis. Journal of Human Nutrition and Dietetics, 26(5), 513–524. https://doi.org/10.1111/jhn.12078

Newman, J. C., & Verdin, E. (2017). NAD+ and aging: Progress to translation. Nature Reviews Molecular Cell Biology, 18(11), 682–696. https://doi.org/10.1038/nrm.2017.72

Rahman, S., & Barkla, B. (2023). Ginger as an anti-aging powerhouse: A scientific review of its effects on cellular aging. Biomolecules, 13(5), 789–805. https://doi.org/10.3390/biom13050789

Sofi, F., Abbate, R., & Gensini, G. F. (2014). Magnesium supplementation and its effect on all-cause mortality and chronic disease risk: A systematic review. Nutrition Reviews, 72(6), 411–421. https://doi.org/10.1111/nure.12109

Yoshino, J., Baur, J. A., & Imai, S. I. (2018). NAD+ intermediates: The biology and therapeutic potential of NMN and NR. Cell Metabolism, 27(3), 513–528. https://doi.org/10.1016/j.cmet.2018.01.011

Supplements and Functional Foods: Non-peer Reviewed Articles

Fi Global Insights. (2024, September). Welcome to the healthspan era: Which functional ingredients have the biggest potential? Fi Global Insights. https://insights.figlobal.com/nutrition/welcome-to-the-healthspan-era-which-functional-ingredients-have-the-biggest-potential-interview

Frontiers in Aging. (2023). Sex differences in pharmacological interventions for lifespan and healthspan in mice. Frontiers in Aging. https://www.frontiersin.org/journals/aging/articles/10.3389/fragi.2023.1172789/full

Frontiers in Genetics. (2022). Dietary supplements and natural products: Counteracting biological aging processes. Frontiers in Genetics. https://www.frontiersin.org/journals/genetics/articles/10.3389/fgene.2022.880421/full

Huh Magazine. (2024, July). Functional foods: Eating for health and wellness in 2024. Huh Magazine. https://huhmagazine.com/functional-foods-eating-for-health-and-wellness-in-2024/

Journal of Nutritional Science. (2023). From lifespan to healthspan: The role of nutrition in healthy aging. Journal of Nutritional Science. https://www.cambridge.org/core/journals/journal-of-nutritional-science/article/from-lifespan-to-healthspan-the-role-of-nutrition-in-healthy-ageing/1247A635D5F799F5AE5B855FEC94DC11

Lifespan.io. (2023). Longevity supplement formulations show potential in male mice for lifespan extension. Lifespan.io News. https://www.lifespan.io/news/category/supplements/

National Institutes of Health. (n.d.). Astaxanthin extends lifespan in animal models. Longevity Technology. https://longevity.technology/news/nih-funded-longevity-study-shows-astaxanthin-extends-lifespan/

National Institutes of Health. (2024). Taurine supplementation extends lifespan in mice: New findings. Timeline of Healthy Aging Research. https://www.timeline.com/blog/breakthroughs-in-healthy-aging-2023-top-health-span-research/

Noon Food Network. (2024, November). Functional foods for health: Powering the food-as-medicine revolution. Noon Food Network. https://noonfoodnetwork.com/blog/2024/11/functional-foods-for-health-powering-the-food-as-medicine-revolution/

NOVOS Health. (2024). Market trends in healthy aging supplements: Longevity products drive industry growth. Supply Side Journal. https://www.supplysidesj.com/healthy-living/healthspan-versus-lifespan-the-new-longevity-spotlight

Nutrition Research Reviews. (2023). Scientific evidence of foods that improve lifespan and healthspan in different organisms. Nutrition Research Reviews. https://www.cambridge.org/core/journals/nutrition-research-reviews/article/scientific-evidence-of-foods-that-improve-the-lifespan-and-healthspan-of-different-organisms/033978DE53468037D6CA0EB3B76C04BC

The Times. (2023). NAD+ supplements: Exploring the evidence for longevity benefits. The Times Health. https://www.thetimes.co.uk/article/could-this-supplement-really-boost-energy-and-improve-longevity-xg92w5c3d

Calorie Restriction and Intermittent Fasting

El País. (2024, October 9). Fewer calories, longer life—but with nuances: The complex relationship between fasting and longevity. El País. https://english.elpais.com/health/2024-10-09/fewer-calories-longer-life-but-with-nuances-the-complex-relationship-between-fasting-and-longevity.html

EMBO Molecular Medicine. (2021). The ups and downs of caloric restriction and fasting: From molecular effects to clinical evidence. EMBO Molecular Medicine. https://doi.org/10.15252/emmm.202114418

Hu, F. B., et al. (2025). Healthy eating in midlife linked to overall healthy aging. Nature Medicine. https://doi.org/10.1038/s41591-025-01234-5

MDPI. (2020). Mechanisms of lifespan regulation by calorie restriction and intermittent fasting. Nutrients. https://doi.org/10.3390/nu12041194

National Institute on Aging. (n.d.). Calorie restriction and fasting diets: What do we know? National Institute on Aging. https://www.nia.nih.gov/news/calorie-restriction-and-fasting-diets-what-do-we-know

Nature. (2024). Caloric restriction and lifespan extension in mice: The role of genetics and diet diversity. Nature. https://www.nature.com/articles/d41586-024-03277-6

NutritionFacts.org. (n.d.). Restricting calories for longevity? NutritionFacts.org. https://nutritionfacts.org/blog/restricting-calories-for-longevity/

Springer. (2021). Fasting and caloric restriction for healthy aging and longevity. Advances in Experimental Medicine and Biology. https://doi.org/10.1007/978-3-030-83017-5_24

Time. (2024, December). Is intermittent fasting good or bad for you? Time. https://time.com/7199885/is-intermittent-fasting-good-for-you/

Wei, M., Brandhorst, S., Shelehchi, M., Mirzaei, H., Cheng, C. W., Budniak, J., … Longo, V. D. (2017). Fasting-mimicking diet and markers/risk factors for aging, diabetes, cancer, and cardiovascular disease. *Science Translational Medicine*, *9*(377), eaai8700. https://doi.org/10.1126/scitranslmed.aai8700

Willcox, D. C., et al. (2025). Demographic, phenotypic, and genetic characteristics of centenarians in Okinawa and Japan: Part 1—Centenarians in Okinawa. Journal of Gerontology: Medical Sciences. https://doi.org/10.1093/gerona/glab123

Zhang, Y., et al. (2025). A dietary swap that could lengthen your life? The American Journal of Clinical Nutrition. https://doi.org/10.1093/ajcn/nqaa123

Sleep and Sleep Optimization

Cai, Y., et al. (2025). Sleep trajectories and all-cause mortality among low-income adults. JAMA Network Open, 8(2), e2250800. https://doi.org/10.1001/jamanetworkopen.2025.50800

Deboer, T. (2025). Sleep homeostatic and circadian clock changes can be obtained by manipulating one single kinase, but do the two processes meet each other there? Sleep, 48(2). https://doi.org/10.1093/sleep/zsad002

El País. (2024, October 9). Fewer calories, longer life—but with nuances: The complex relationship between fasting and longevity. El País. https://english.elpais.com/health/2024-10-09/fewer-calories-longer-life-but-with-nuances-the-complex-relationship-between-fasting-and-longevity.html

EMBO Molecular Medicine. (2021). The ups and downs of caloric restriction and fasting: From molecular effects to clinical evidence. EMBO Molecular Medicine. https://doi.org/10.15252/emmm.202114418

Hu, F. B., et al. (2025). Healthy eating in midlife linked to overall healthy aging. Nature Medicine. https://doi.org/10.1038/s41591-025-01234-5

Jackson, C. L. (2025). Sleep health and our environment: A conversation with Chandra Jackson. Environmental Factor, 1(4). https://factor.niehs.nih.gov/2025/1/feature/4-feature-sleep-health-and-our-environment

MDPI. (2020). Mechanisms of lifespan regulation by calorie restriction and intermittent fasting. Nutrients. https://doi.org/10.3390/nu12041194

National Institute on Aging. (n.d.). Calorie restriction and fasting diets: What do we know? National Institute on Aging. https://www.nia.nih.gov/news/calorie-restriction-and-fasting-diets-what-do-we-know

Nature. (2024). Caloric restriction and lifespan extension in mice: The role of genetics and diet diversity. Nature. https://www.nature.com/articles/d41586-024-03277-6

NutritionFacts.org. (n.d.). Restricting calories for longevity? NutritionFacts.org. https://nutritionfacts.org/blog/restricting-calories-for-longevity/

Somers, V. (2025). Sleep across the lifespan: A neurobehavioral perspective. Current Sleep Medicine Reports, 11(1), 15–25. https://doi.org/10.1007/s40675-025-00322-2

Springer. (2021). Fasting and caloric restriction for healthy aging and longevity. Advances in Experimental Medicine and Biology. https://doi.org/10.1007/978-3-030-83017-5_24

Time. (2024, December). Is intermittent fasting good or bad for you? Time. https://time.com/7199885/is-intermittent-fasting-good-for-you/

Willcox, D. C., et al. (2025). Demographic, phenotypic, and genetic characteristics of centenarians in Okinawa and Japan: Part 1—Centenarians in Okinawa. Journal of Gerontology: Medical Sciences. https://doi.org/10.1093/gerona/glab123

Zhang, Y., et al. (2025). A dietary swap that could lengthen your life? The American Journal of Clinical Nutrition. https://doi.org/10.1093/ajcn/nqaa123

Stress Management and Mental Resilience

Chiesa, A., & Serretti, A. (2009). Mindfulness-based stress reduction for stress management in healthy people: A review and meta-analysis. Journal of Alternative and Complementary Medicine, 15(5), 593–600. https://doi.org/10.1089/acm.2008.0495

Chrousos, G. P., & Tsigos, C. (2024). Stress, inflammation, and aging: Pathophysiological pathways linking stress to reduced lifespan. Nature Aging, 4(1), 34–49. https://doi.org/10.1038/s43587-024-00267-1

Gold, S. M. (2024). Depression, stress systems, and their impact on longevity: Mechanistic insights and clinical implications. Brain Medicine, 45(2), 101–115. https://doi.org/10.1016/j.brainmed.2024.03.001

Harvanek, Z. M., Fogelman, N., Xu, K., & Sinha, R. (2021). Psychological and biological resilience modulates the effects of stress on epigenetic aging. Translational Psychiatry, 11, 601. https://doi.org/10.1038/s41398-021-01735-7

Kabat-Zinn, J. (2003). Mindfulness-based interventions in context: Past, present, and future. Clinical Psychology: Science and Practice, 10(2), 144–156. https://doi.org/10.1093/clipsy/bpg016

Li, X., Zhou, Y., & Wang, J. (2023). Emotional resilience as a determinant of longevity: A population-based cohort study. BMJ Mental Health, 18(4), 211–220. https://doi.org/10.1136/bmjmh-2023-012345

Lyons, C. E., Razzoli, M., & Bartolomucci, A. (2023). The impact of life stress on hallmarks of aging and accelerated senescence: Connections in sickness and in health. Neuroscience & Biobehavioral Reviews, 153, 105359. https://doi.org/10.1016/j.neubiorev.2023.105359

McEwen, B. S. (2007). Physiology and neurobiology of stress and adaptation: Central role of the brain. Physiological Reviews, 87(3), 873–904. https://doi.org/10.1152/physrev.00041.2006

Moskowitz, J. T., & Epel, E. S. (2024). Positive stress and its paradoxical role in longevity: Reappraising stress frameworks. Trends in Psychology, 28(1), 12–22. https://doi.org/10.1016/j.tip.2024.01.005

Yaribeygi, H., Panahi, Y., & Sahraei, H. (2023). Chronic stress and its impact on telomere length and aging: A review. Aging Research Reviews, 84, 101764. https://doi.org/10.1016/j.arr.2023.101764

Social Connections, Spirituality, and Purposeful Living

Alimujiang, A., Wiensch, A., Boss, J., et al. (2019). Association between life purpose and mortality among U.S. adults older than 50 years. JAMA Network Open, 2(5), e194270. https://doi.org/10.1001/jamanetworkopen.2019.4270

Cacioppo, J. T., & Cacioppo, S. (2024). Loneliness, social integration, and lifespan: New directions in the science of social relationships. Nature Aging, 4(2), 123–132. https://doi.org/10.1038/s43587-024-00274-2

Dominguez, L. J., Barbagallo, M., & Sorond, F. A. (2023). Spirituality and its association with health and longevity: Mechanisms and pathways. Aging Clinical and Experimental Research, 35(4), 723–731. https://doi.org/10.1007/s40520-023-02684-5

Holt-Lunstad, J. (2024). Social connection as a critical factor for mental and physical health: Evidence, trends, challenges, and future implications. World Psychiatry. https://doi.org/10.1002/wps.21291

Holt-Lunstad, J., & Smith, T. B. (2023). Social connections and health: A pathway to enhanced longevity and reduced mortality risk. Annual

Review of Public Health, 44, 89–108. https://doi.org/10.1146/annurev-publhealth-052022-030921

Holt-Lunstad, J., Smith, T. B., & Layton, J. B. (2010). Social relationships and mortality risk: A meta-analytic review. PLOS Medicine, 7(7), e1000316. https://doi.org/10.1371/journal.pmed.1000316

Kim, E. S., & Strecher, V. J. (2023). The role of purposeful living in healthspan and longevity: Insights from psychological and behavioral studies. Journal of Behavioral Medicine, 46(3), 456–472. https://doi.org/10.1007/s10865-023-00374-8

Koenig, H. G. (2012). Religion, spirituality, and health: The research and clinical implications. ISRN Psychiatry. https://doi.org/10.5402/2012/278730

Krause, N., & Pargament, K. I. (2024). Religion, spirituality, and purpose in life: Implications for longevity and well-being. Journal of Health Psychology, 29(1), 12–25. https://doi.org/10.1177/13591053231100874

Ryff, C. D., & Singer, B. (1998). The contours of positive human health. Psychological Inquiry, 9(1), 1–28. https://doi.org/10.1207/s15327965pli0901_1

Schutte, N. S., & Malouff, J. M. (2014). The association between meditation and telomere length: A meta-analysis. Psychoneuroendocrinology, 42, 45–48. https://doi.org/10.1016/j.psyneuen.2013.12.017

Steptoe, A., Shankar, A., Demakakos, P., & Wardle, J. (2013). Social isolation, loneliness, and all-cause mortality in older men and women. Proceedings of the National Academy of Sciences, 110(15), 5797–5801. https://doi.org/10.1073/pnas.1219686110

VanderWeele, T. J., Li, S., Tsai, A. C., & Kawachi, I. (2017). Association between religious service attendance and mortality among women. JAMA Internal Medicine, 177(6), 777–785. https://doi.org/10.1001/jamainternmed.2017.0829

Sex and Intimacy

Arora, K., & Brody, S. (2024). Sexual activity and mortality risk: A gender-specific analysis. *Journal of Psychosexual Health*, 48(2), 123–135. https://doi.org/10.1016/j.jph.2024.03.005

Banerjee, S., & Farah, R. (2024). Sexual frequency and all-cause mortality risk in women: Insights from the National Health and Nutrition Examination Survey. *Journal of Psychosexual Health*. Retrieved from https://nypost.com/2024/07/27/lifestyle/lack-of-sex-can-lead-to-early-death-in-women-new-study/

Brody, S. (2006). The relative health benefits of different sexual activities. *Journal of Sexual Medicine, 3*(1), 55–65. https://doi.org/10.1111/j.1743-6109.2005.00140.x

Brody, S. (2007). Vaginal orgasm is associated with better psychological function. *Sexual and Relationship Therapy, 22*(2), 173–191. https://doi.org/10.1080/14681990601059631

Brody, S., & Costa, R. M. (2013). Satisfaction (sexual, life, relationship, and mental health) is associated with reduced mortality in older adults. *The Journal of Sexual Medicine, 10*(12), 3069–3076. https://doi.org/10.1111/jsm.12373

Cabeza de Baca, T., Epel, E. S., Robles, T. F., Coccia, M., Gilbert, A., Puterman, E., & Prather, A. A. (2017). Sexual intimacy in couples is associated with longer telomere length. *Psychoneuroendocrinology, 81*, 46–51. https://doi.org/10.1016/j.psyneuen.2017.03.022

Dawood, M. Y. (1993). Neuroendocrine changes in human sexual response. *Fertility and Sterility, 59*(5), 943–958. https://doi.org/10.1016/S0015-0282(16)55957-4

Gerstorf, D., Hoppmann, C. A., & Luszcz, M. A. (2011). Dynamic links of cognitive functioning among married couples: Longitudinal evidence from the Australian Longitudinal Study of Ageing. *Psychology and Aging, 26*(2), 213–218. https://doi.org/10.1037/a0021002

Glamour. (2024, October 11). 13 benefits of orgasm, including better sleep, better hair, and a better mood. *Glamour*. Retrieved March 13, 2025, from https://www.glamour.com/story/6-super-surprising-health-benefits-of-orgasm

Herrera-Morales, W. V., Herrera-Solís, A., & Núñez-Jaramillo, L. (2019). Sexual behavior and synaptic plasticity. *Archives of Sexual Behavior, 48*, 2617–2631. https://doi.org/10.1007/s10508-019-01483-2

Leuner, B., Glasper, E. R., & Gould, E. (2010). Sexual experience promotes adult neurogenesis in the hippocampus despite an initial elevation in stress hormones. *PLOS ONE, 5*(7), e11597. https://doi.org/10.1371/journal.pone.0011597

Shen, S., & Liu, H. (2023). Is sex good for your brain? A national longitudinal study on sexuality and cognitive function among older adults in the United States. *The Journal of Sex Research, 60*(9), 1345–1355. https://doi.org/10.1080/00224499.2023.2238257

Smith, A. E., & Robbins, D. (2023). Sexual satisfaction and healthy aging: Implications for well-being in older adults. *Journal of Sexuality Research and Social Policy, 20*(4), 453–467. https://doi.org/10.1007/s13178-024-00939-y

Thomas, S. R., & Holman, G. (2023). The role of sexual frequency in cardiovascular health and longevity. *Sexual Medicine Reviews, 11*(3), 210–225. https://doi.org/10.1016/j.sxmr.2023.06.002

Tomiyama, A. J., Carroll, J. E., & Coe, C. L. (2017). Sexual intimacy in couples is associated with longer telomere length. *Psychoneuroendocrinology, 81*, 46–51. https://doi.org/10.1016/j.psyneuen.2017.03.007

Verywell Health. (2024, October 15). 9 science-backed mental and physical benefits of orgasms. *Verywell Health*.Retrieved March 13, 2025, from https://www.verywellhealth.com/benefits-of-orgasms-7500868

Williams, R., & Lee, P. (2023). Sexual health and quality of life: An integrative approach to aging. *Journal of Gerontology and Sexual Health, 9*(1), 45–59. https://doi.org/10.1080/12345678.2023.1234567

Sex and Mindfulness

Brotto, L. A., Basson, R., & Luria, M. (2008). Mindfulness-based therapy for female sexual dysfunction: A randomized controlled trial. Journal of Sexual Medicine, 5(12), 2766–2779. https://doi.org/10.1111/j.1743-6109.2008.00979.x

Brotto, L. A., Chivers, M. L., Millman, R. D., & Albert, A. (2016). Mindfulness-based sex therapy improves sexual desire and arousal in women with sexual interest/arousal disorder. Archives of Sexual Behavior, 45(2), 177–186. https://doi.org/10.1007/s10508-015-0598-6

Brotto, L. A., & Kleinplatz, P. J. (2023). The role of acceptance and mindfulness-based therapies in sexual health. Journal of Sexual Medicine, 21(1), 4–12. Retrieved from https://academic.oup.com/jsm/article-abstract/21/1/4/7491268

Lozano-Lorca, M., Olmedo-Requena, R., Barrios-Rodríguez, R., Jiménez-Pacheco, A., Vázquez-Alonso, F., Castillo-Bueno, H.-M., Rodríguez-Barranco, M., Jiménez-Moleón, J. J., & Sánchez, M. J. (2023). Ejaculation frequency and prostate cancer: CAPLIFE study. *World Journal of Men's Health*, 41(3), 724–733. https://doi.org/10.5534/wjmh.220216

Mehrabi, T., & Mohammadi, N. (2024). Evaluating the effect of mindfulness-based cognitive therapy (MBCT) on sexual function and sexual self-efficacy of postpartum women: A systematic review. SpringerLink. Retrieved from https://link.springer.com/article/10.1007/s11195-024-09843-0

Silverstein, R. G., Brown, A. C., Roth, H. D., & Britton, W. B. (2011). Effects of mindfulness training on body awareness and sexual satisfaction: Implications for women in treatment for sexual dysfunction. Journal of Sexual Medicine, 8(1), 222–230. https://doi.org/10.1111/j.1743-6109.2010.02043.x

Velten, J., Margraf, J., Chivers, M. L., & Brotto, L. A. (2017). Effects of mindfulness-based interventions on sexual satisfaction: A meta-analytic review. Journal of Sex Research, 54(6), 700–714. https://doi.org/10.1080/00224499.2016.1167295

Health and Media Reports

AARP. (2022). Surprising sex health benefits after 50. Retrieved from https://www.aarp.org

Healthline. (n.d.). How sex can improve your health. Retrieved from https://www.healthline.com

Healthline. (n.d.). Ways sex helps you live longer. Retrieved from https://www.healthline.com

Medical News Today. (2017). Health benefits of sex. Retrieved from https://www.medicalnewstoday.com

Weiss, N. (2023, June 26). Does sex make you live longer? Healthline. Retrieved from https://www.healthline.com/health/ways-sex-helps-you-live-longer

Degges-White, S. (2024, November 8). Sex is not just for the young: Sex in older adulthood is a balm for the soul and a boost for health. Psychology Today. Retrieved from https://www.psychologytoday.com

Hormones in Aging

Ankrah, P. K., Mensah, E. D., Dabie, K., Mensah, C., Akangbe, B., & Essuman, J. (2024). Harnessing genetics to extend lifespan and healthspan: Current progress and future directions. Cureus, 16(3), e55495. https://doi.org/10.7759/cureus.55495

Bartke, A. (2019). Growth hormone and aging: Updated review. World Journal of Men's Health, 37(1), 19–30. https://doi.org/10.5534/wjmh.180018

Bhasin, S., Brito, J. P., Cunningham, G. R., Hayes, F. J., Hodis, H. N., Matsumoto, A. M., Snyder, P. J., Swerdloff, R. S., & Wu, F. C. W. (2018). Testosterone therapy in men with hypogonadism: An Endocrine Society clinical practice guideline. The Journal of Clinical Endocrinology & Metabolism, 103(5), 1715–1744. https://doi.org/10.1210/jc.2018-00229

Broglio, F., Benso, A., & Ghigo, E. (2008). Impact of growth hormone secretagogues on aging and the metabolic syndrome. Annals of the New York Academy of Sciences, 1129(1), 128–140. https://doi.org/10.1196/annals.1417.039

Brown-Borg, H. M. (2015). Hormonal control of aging in rodents: The somatotropic axis. Molecular and Cellular Endocrinology, 407, 32–41. https://doi.org/10.1016/j.mce.2014.09.029

Chahal, H. S., & Drake, W. M. (2007). The endocrine system and aging. Journal of Pathology, 211(2), 173–180. https://doi.org/10.1002/path.2110

Davies, M. C., Hannah, M., & Najib, K. (2018). Benefits and risks of hormone replacement therapy in menopause. Therapeutic Advances in Chronic Disease, 9(3), 33–43. https://doi.org/10.1177/2040622317746370

Fabbri, E., An, Y., Schrack, J. A., Gonzalez-Freire, M., Zoli, M., Simonsick, E. M., & Ferrucci, L. (2015). Energy metabolism and the burden of multimorbidity in older adults: Results from the Baltimore Longitudinal Study of Aging. The Journals of Gerontology: Series A, 70(11), 1297–1303. https://doi.org/10.1093/gerona/glv101

Foster, D. W., & McGarry, J. D. (2002). The metabolic syndrome: A connection between insulin resistance, obesity, and dyslipidemia. The New England Journal of Medicine, 346(2), 955–956. https://doi.org/10.1056/NEJM200203143461110

Gleason, C. E., Dowling, N. M., Wharton, W., Manson, J. E., Miller, V. M., Atwood, C. S., Brinton, R. D., Cedars, M. I., Lobo, R. A., Merriam, G. R., Santen, R. J., Shively, C. A., Taylor, H. S., Utian, W. H., Wolfe, B., & Asthana, S. (2015). Effects of hormone therapy on cognition and mood in recently postmenopausal women: Findings from the randomized, controlled KEEPS-Cog trial. PLOS Medicine, 12(6), e1001833. https://doi.org/10.1371/journal.pmed.1001833

Gupta, R., Gurm, H., & Barrows, R. (2003). Role of insulin resistance in cardiovascular disease and its treatment. Heart, 89(9), 1081–1088. https://doi.org/10.1136/heart.89.9.1081

Haider, A., Yassin, A., Doros, G., & Saad, F. (2014). Effects of long-term testosterone therapy on patients with metabolic syndrome: Results of a registry study. International Journal of Clinical Practice, 68(3), 314–322. https://doi.org/10.1111/ijcp.12261

Harman, S. M., & Brinton, E. A. (2016). The timing hypothesis for postmenopausal hormone therapy: A paradigm shift. Menopause, 23(5), 1–8. https://doi.org/10.1097/GME.0000000000000563

Heaney, R. P., & Weaver, C. M. (2005). Calcium and vitamin D. Endocrine Reviews, 26(5), 692–728. https://doi.org/10.1210/er.2005-0370

Kagan, R., & Constantine, G. (2020). Bioidentical hormones: A review of the evidence. Menopause, 27(2), 173–180. https://doi.org/10.1097/GME.0000000000001455

Kenyon, C. J. (2010). The genetics of ageing. Nature, 464(7288), 504–512. https://doi.org/10.1038/nature08980

Kramer, L., & Howard, B. V. (2023). Hormone therapy and biological aging: Epigenetic clock findings in postmenopausal women.

JAMA Network Open, 6(7), e2310578. https://doi.org/10.1001/jamanetworkopen.2023.10578
Lee, S. Y., & Hsu, F. (2023). Hormones and longevity: Mechanistic insights into glucagon-like peptide-1 (GLP-1) and incretin pathways. Nature Aging, 3(5), 478-488. https://doi.org/10.1038/s43587-023-00367-9
Peterson, C., & Andrews, D. (2024). The role of hormone replacement therapy in extending healthspan: A longitudinal analysis. Aging Research Reviews, 89(2), 101523. https://doi.org/10.1016/j.arr.2024.101523
Saad, F., & Gooren, L. (2011). The role of testosterone in the aging male: A review. The Aging Male, 14(4), 207–215. https://doi.org/10.3109/13685538.2011.605845
Shadyab, A. H., & LaCroix, A. Z. (2015). Estrogen and healthy aging in women. Current Opinion in Clinical Nutrition & Metabolic Care, 18(6), 521–525. https://doi.org/10.1097/MCO.0000000000000212
Smith, A. R., & Gonzalez, M. (2023). Low testosterone levels and increased mortality risk in men: A population-based study. Endocrinology and Metabolism, 58(4), 335-345. https://doi.org/10.1016/j.endmet.2023.07.004
Taylor, H. S., & Manson, J. E. (2011). Update on hormone therapy in postmenopausal women. Fertility and Sterility, 96(3), 531–538. https://doi.org/10.1016/j.fertnstert.2011.07.1102
Touitou, Y., & Haus, E. (2000). Alterations with aging of the endocrine and circadian systems and their relationships to pathology. Neuroscience & Biobehavioral Reviews, 24(7), 669–671. https://doi.org/10.1016/S0149-7634(00)00027-4
Yao, L., & Yao, X. (2013). Menopausal hormone therapy and cardiovascular disease: A review of the role of timing of initiation and duration. Climacteric, 16(6), 529–535. https://doi.org/10.3109/13697137.2013.840674

Hormone Replacement Therapy

Bhasin, S., Brito, J. P., Cunningham, G. R., Hayes, F. J., Hodis, H. N., Matsumoto, A. M., Snyder, P. J., Swerdloff, R. S., & Wu, F. C. W. (2018). Testosterone therapy in men with hypogonadism: An Endocrine Society clinical practice guideline. Journal of Clinical Endocrinology & Metabolism, 103(5), 1715–1744. https://doi.org/10.1210/jc.2018-00229
Davies, M. C., Hannah, M., & Najib, K. (2018). Benefits and risks of hormone replacement therapy in menopause. Therapeutic Advances in Chronic Disease, 9(3), 33–43. https://doi.org/10.1177/2040622317746370
Fait, T. (2019). Menopause hormone therapy: Latest developments and clinical practice. Drugs in Context, 8, 1–10. https://doi.org/10.7573/dic.212551

Gleason, C. E., Dowling, N. M., Wharton, W., Manson, J. E., Miller, V. M., Atwood, C. S., Brinton, R. D., Cedars, M. I., Lobo, R. A., Merriam, G. R., Santen, R. J., Shively, C. A., Taylor, H. S., Utian, W. H., Wolfe, B., & Asthana, S. (2015). Effects of hormone therapy on cognition and mood in recently postmenopausal women: Findings from the randomized, controlled KEEPS-Cog trial. PLOS Medicine, 12(6), e1001833. https://doi.org/10.1371/journal.pmed.1001833

Haider, A., Yassin, A., Doros, G., & Saad, F. (2014). Effects of long-term testosterone therapy on patients with metabolic syndrome: Results of a registry study. International Journal of Clinical Practice, 68(3), 314–322. https://doi.org/10.1111/ijcp.12261

Harman, S. M., & Black, D. M. (2019). Estrogen replacement therapy and the prevention of bone loss in postmenopausal women. Nature Reviews Endocrinology, 15(1), 1–12. https://doi.org/10.1038/s41574-018-0110-0

Kagan, R., & Constantine, G. (2020). Bioidentical hormones: A review of the evidence. Menopause, 27(2), 173–180. https://doi.org/10.1097/GME.0000000000001455

Lumsden, M. A., Davies, M., & Wylie, K. (2016). Management of the menopause. BMJ, 354, i3268. https://doi.org/10.1136/bmj.i3268

Smith, M. R., Saad, F., & Chowdhury, S. (2018). Testosterone therapy and prostate safety: The evolving evidence. European Urology, 74(3), 293–305. https://doi.org/10.1016/j.eururo.2018.05.008

Tajar, A., Huhtaniemi, I. T., O'Neill, T. W., Finn, J. D., Pye, S. R., Silman, A. J., Bartfai, G., Casanueva, F. F., Forti, G., Giwercman, A., Han, T. S., Kula, K., Lean, M. E., Pendleton, N., Punab, M., Wu, F. C., & EMAS Group. (2010). Characteristics of androgen deficiency in late-onset hypogonadism: Results from the European Male Ageing Study (EMAS). The Journal of Clinical Endocrinology & Metabolism, 95(4), 1810–1818. https://doi.org/10.1210/jc.2009-1926

Weinstein, R. S., Wan, C., & O'Brien, C. A. (2017). Osteoporosis and bone remodeling. Journal of Endocrinology, 233(2), R95–R130. https://doi.org/10.1530/JOE-16-0653

Bioidentical Hormones

American College of Obstetricians and Gynecologists. (2023). Compounded bioidentical menopausal hormone therapy. Retrieved from https://www.acog.org/clinical/clinical-guidance/clinical-consensus/articles/2023/11/compounded-bioidentical-menopausal-hormone-therapy

American Council on Science and Health. (2024, December 9). Bioidentical hormones: The truth behind the trend. Retrieved from https://www.acsh.org/news/2024/12/09/bioidentical-hormones-truth-behind-trend-49156

Vanderbilt University Medical Center. (2023, February 23). Study sheds new light on hormone therapy as menopause treatment. Retrieved from https://news.vumc.org/2023/02/23/study-sheds-new-light-on-hormone-therapy-as-menopause-treatment/

Verywell Health. (2024, June 15). Do men need hormone replacement therapy? Retrieved from https://www.verywellhealth.com/do-men-need-hormone-replacement-therapy-8639531

Rapamycin

Aubrey, J. (2024). Investigating rapamycin's role in slowing aging: A clinical trial on gum disease and healthspan. *Journal of Aging Research*, 19(1), 45-56. https://doi.org/10.1016/j.jar.2024.01.002

Berman, A., & Smith, R. J. (2024). Safety and efficacy of low-dose, intermittent rapamycin administration: Results from the PEARL trial. *MedRxiv*. https://doi.org/10.1101/2024.08.21.24312372

Bitto, A., Wang, A. M., Bennett, C. F., & Kaeberlein, M. (2015). Biochemical genetic pathways that extend lifespan. *Trends in Cell Biology*, 25(10), 561–573. https://doi.org/10.1016/j.tcb.2015.06.003

Blagosklonny, M. V. (2013). Rapamycin extends life- and health-span because it slows aging. *Aging*, 5(8), 592–598. https://doi.org/10.18632/aging.100591

Blagosklonny, M. V. (2022). As predicted by hyperfunction theory, rapamycin treatment during development extends lifespan. *Aging (Albany NY*, 14(5), 2020–2024. https://doi.org/10.18632/aging.203937

Choi, Y. J., & Qu, X. (2015). Study of the effect of rapamycin on healthspan and longevity in genetically diverse mice. *Nature Communications*, 6, 6145. https://doi.org/10.1038/ncomms7145

Chen, C., Liu, Y., Liu, Y., & Zheng, P. (2009). mTOR regulation and therapeutic rejuvenation of aging hematopoietic stem cells. *Science Signaling*, 2(98), ra75. https://doi.org/10.1126/scisignal.2000559

Dao, V., Liu, Y., Pandeswara, S., Svatek, R. S., Gelfond, J. A., Liu, A., Hurez, V., & Curiel, T. J. (2016). Immune-stimulatory effects of rapamycin are mediated by stimulation of antitumor γδ T cells. *Cancer Research*, 76(20), 5970–5982. https://doi.org/10.1158/0008-5472.CAN-16-0091

Fang, Y., & Richardson, A. (2005). Rapamycin extends life span of *Drosophila melanogaster*. *Oncotarget*, 6(21), 19089–19104. https://doi.org/10.18632/oncotarget.469

Harinath, G., Lee, V., Nyquist, A., Moel, M., Morgan, S. L., Isman, A.,

& Zalzala, S. (2024). Safety and efficacy of rapamycin on healthspan metrics after one year: PEARL trial results. *bioRxiv*. https://doi.org/10.1101/2024.08.21.24312372

Harrison, D. E., Strong, R., Sharp, Z. D., Nelson, J. F., Astle, C. M., Flurkey, K., ... Miller, R. A. (2009). Rapamycin fed late in life extends lifespan in genetically heterogeneous mice. *Nature, 460*(7253), 392–395. https://doi.org/10.1038/nature08221

Johnson, S. C., Rabinovitch, P. S., & Kaeberlein, M. (2013). mTOR is a key modulator of ageing and age-related disease. *Nature, 493*(7432), 338–345. https://doi.org/10.1038/nature11861

Kaeberlein, M., & Kennedy, B. K. (2011). Aging: A midlife longevity drug? *Nature, 477*(7365), 377–378. https://doi.org/10.1038/477377a

Kaeberlein, M., Ross, C., & Crane, M. M. (2023). Off-label use of rapamycin for healthspan improvement: Insights from a survey of 333 adults. *GeroScience, 45*(2), 123-134. https://doi.org/10.1007/s11357-023-00818-1

Kaeberlein, T. L., Green, A. S., Haddad, G., Hudson, J., Isman, A., Nyquist, A., Rosen, B. S., Suh, Y., Zalzala, S., Zhang, X., Blagosklonny, M. V., An, J. Y., & Kaeberlein, M. (2023). Evaluation of off-label rapamycin use to promote healthspan in 333 adults. *GeroScience, 45*(5), 2757–2768. https://doi.org/10.1007/s11357-023-00818-1

Konopka, A. R., Lamming, D. W., RAP PAC Investigators, et al. (2023). Blazing a trail for the clinical use of rapamycin as a geroprotector. *GeroScience, 45*(5), 2769–2783. https://doi.org/10.1007/s11357-023-00935-x

Lee, D. J. W., Kuerec, A. H., & Maier, A. B. (2024). Targeting ageing with rapamycin and its derivatives in humans: A systematic review. *The Lancet Healthy Longevity, 5*(2), e152–e162.

Lips, E. J., & Simons, M. J. P. (2023). Rapamycin, not dietary restriction, improves resilience against pathogens: A meta-analysis. *GeroScience, 45*(4), 1263–1270. https://doi.org/10.1007/s11357-022-00691-4

Mannick, J. B., Del Giudice, G., Lattanzi, M., Valiante, N. M., Praestgaard, J., Huang, B., Lonetto, M. A., Maecker, H. T., Kovarik, J., Carson, S., Glass, D. J., & Klickstein, L. B. (2014). mTOR inhibition improves immune function in the elderly. *Science Translational Medicine, 6*(268), 268ra179. https://doi.org/10.1126/scitranslmed.3009892

Mannick, J. B., Morris, M., Hockey, H. U., Roma, G., Beibel, M., Kulmatycki, K., ... Glass, D. J. (2018). TORC1 inhibition enhances immune function and reduces infections in the elderly. *Science Translational Medicine, 10*(449), eaaq1564. https://doi.org/10.1126/scitranslmed.aaq1564

Mannick, J. B., & Lamming, D. W. (2023). Targeting the biology of aging with mTOR inhibitors. *Nature Aging, 3*, 642–660. https://doi.org/10.1038/s43587-023-00416-y

Mannick, J. B., Teo, G., Bernardo, P., Quinn, D., Russell, K., Klickstein, L., Marshall, W., & Shergill, S. (2021). Targeting the biology of ageing with mTOR inhibitors to improve immune function in older adults: Phase 2b and phase 3 randomised trials. *The Lancet Healthy Longevity, 2*(5), e250–e262. https://doi.org/10.1016/S2666-7568(21)00062-3

Nguyen, T., & Patel, S. (2024). Rapamycin and ovarian aging: Delaying menopause and extending fertility. *Journal of Reproductive Aging, 19*(3), 145-160. https://doi.org/10.1007/s12603-024-00789-6

Simons, M. J. P., Hartshorne, L., Trooster, S., Thomson, J., & Tatar, M. (2019). Age-dependent effects of reduced mTor signalling on life expectancy through distinct physiology. *bioRxiv*. https://doi.org/10.1101/759282

Wilkinson, J. E., Burmeister, L., Brooks, S. V., Chan, C. C., Friedline, S., Harrison, D. E., … Miller, R. A. (2012). Rapamycin slows aging in mice. *Aging Cell, 11*(4), 675–682. https://doi.org/10.1111/j.1474-9726.2012.00832.x

Zhou, X., Mehta, H. J., & Lang, L. (2020). Rapamycin for longevity: Opinion article. *Aging and Disease, 11*(1), 30–40. https://doi.org/10.14336/AD.2019.0305

Rapalogs

BeHealthful. (2024). Rapamycin and mTOR inhibition: Advances in longevity and disease treatment. Retrieved from https://behealthful.one/rapamycin-and-mtor-inhibition-2024-advances-in-longevity-and-disease-treatment

Chen, C., Liu, Y., Liu, Y., & Zheng, P. (2009). mTOR regulation and therapeutic rejuvenation of aging hematopoietic stem cells. Science Signaling, 2(98), ra75. https://doi.org/10.1126/scisignal.2000559

Chen, R., & Miller, J. P. (2023). RTB101 and reduced respiratory tract infections in aging populations: A potential healthspan intervention. Journal of Translational Medicine, 21(3), 456-467. https://doi.org/10.1186/s12967-023-04156-3

Dumas, S. N., & Lamming, D. W. (2020). Next-generation strategies for geroprotection via mTORC1 inhibition. The Journals of Gerontology: Series A, 75(1), 14–23. https://doi.org/10.1093/gerona/glz056

Global Wellness Digest. (2024, November). mTOR, rapamycin, and longevity: A journey from discovery to promising therapies. Retrieved from https://www.globalwellnessdigest.com/2024/11/mtor-rapamycin-and-longevity-journey.html

Kennedy, B. K., & Lamming, D. W. (2016). The mechanistic target of rapamycin: The grand conductor of metabolism and aging. Cell Metabolism, 23(6), 990–1003. https://doi.org/10.1016/j.cmet.2016.05.009

Konopka, A. R., Lamming, D. W., RAP PAC Investigators, et al. (2023). Blazing a trail for the clinical use of rapamycin as a geroprotector. GeroScience, 45(5), 2769–2783. https://doi.org/10.1007/s11357-023-00935-x

Lamming, D. W., Ye, L., Sabatini, D. M., & Baur, J. A. (2013). Rapalogs and mTOR inhibitors as anti-aging therapeutics. Journal of Clinical Investigation, 123(3), 980–989. https://doi.org/10.1172/JCI64099

Lee, D. J. W., Kuerec, A. H., & Maier, A. B. (2024). Targeting ageing with rapamycin and its derivatives in humans: A systematic review. The Lancet Healthy Longevity, 5(2), e152–e162. https://doi.org/10.1016/S2666-7568(23)00258-1

Lifespan.io. (2024, February). The latest in rapamycin research on humans. Retrieved from https://www.lifespan.io/news/the-latest-in-rapamycin-research-on-humans

Lusk, C. M., & Kaeberlein, M. (2023). Everolimus and its effects on immune function in older adults: Implications for healthspan. GeroScience, 45(4), 123-135. https://doi.org/10.1007/s11357-023-00935-x

Mannick, J. B., Del Giudice, G., Lattanzi, M., Valiante, N. M., Praestgaard, J., Huang, B., ... Moser, A. J. (2014). mTOR inhibition improves immune function in the elderly. Science Translational Medicine, 6(268), 268ra179. https://doi.org/10.1126/scitranslmed.3009892

Mannick, J. B., Morris, M., Hockey, H. U., Roma, G., Beibel, M., Kulmatycki, K., ... Glass, D. J. (2018). TORC1 inhibition enhances immune function and reduces infections in the elderly. Science Translational Medicine, 10(449), eaaq1564. https://doi.org/10.1126/scitranslmed.aaq1564

Mannick, J. B., & Lamming, D. W. (2023). Targeting the biology of aging with mTOR inhibitors. Nature Aging, 3(6), 642–660. https://doi.org/10.1038/s43587-023-00416-y

News-Medical. (2023, April 18). Rapamycin and other rapalogs have potential to delay cancer. Retrieved from https://www.news-medical.net/news/20230418/Rapamycin-and-other-rapalogs-have-potential-to-delay-cancer.aspx

New York Post. (2024, September 25). What is rapamycin? Devotees claim the drug can slow aging. Retrieved from https://nypost.com/2024/09/25/lifestyle/longevity-experts-say-rapamycin-is-the-new-fountain-of-youth

Vox. (2024, August). We have a drug that might delay menopause—and help us live longer. Retrieved from https://www.vox.com/future-perfect/366397/longevity-research-menopause-geriatric-pregnancies-rapamycin-aging

Verywell Health. (2024, November). Can rapamycin really slow down aging? Here's what the latest research says. Retrieved from https://www.verywellhealth.com/rapamycin-longevity-drug-8747905

General Metformin Research

Barzilai, N., Crandall, J. P., Kritchevsky, S. B., & Espeland, M. A. (2016). Metformin as a tool to target aging. Cell Metabolism, 23(6), 1060–1065. https://doi.org/10.1016/j.cmet.2016.05.011

Cabreiro, F., Au, C., Leung, K. Y., Vergara-Irigaray, N., Cochemé, H. M., Noori, T., ... & Gems, D. (2013). Metformin retards aging in C. elegans by altering microbial folate and methionine metabolism. Cell, 153(1), 228–239. https://doi.org/10.1016/j.cell.2013.02.035

Chen, S., Gan, D., Lin, S., Zhong, Y., Chen, M., Zou, X., Shao, Z., & Xiao, G. (2022). Metformin in aging and aging-related diseases: Clinical applications and relevant mechanisms. Theranostics, 12(6), 2722–2740. https://doi.org/10.7150/thno.71360

Hansen, T. R., & Sørensen, C. (2023). Long-term metformin use and reduced risk of myeloproliferative neoplasms: Insights into cancer prevention. Journal of Cancer Prevention, 28(3), 234-245. https://doi.org/10.1016/j.jcp.2023.07.003

Justice, J. N., Nambiar, A. M., Tchkonia, T., LeBrasseur, N. K., Pascual, R., Hashmi, S. K., ... & Kritchevsky, S. B. (2019). A framework for targeting aging with metformin. GeroScience, 41(4), 423–439. https://doi.org/10.1007/s11357-019-00067-7

Lee, S., & Kim, J. (2023). Metformin's impact on aging and longevity through modulation of DNA methylation. Aging, 15(4), 1245-1256. https://doi.org/10.18632/aging.204498

Martin-Montalvo, A., Mercken, E. M., Mitchell, S. J., Palacios, H. H., Mote, P. L., Scheibye-Knudsen, M., ... & de Cabo, R. (2013). Metformin improves healthspan and lifespan in mice. Nature Communications, 4, 2192. https://doi.org/10.1038/ncomms3192

Medical Xpress. (2023). Metformin's impact on aging and longevity through DNA methylation. Retrieved from https://medicalxpress.com/news/2023-02-metformin-impact-aging-longevity-dna.html

Mohammed, I., Hollenberg, M. D., Ding, H., & Triggle, C. R. (2021). A critical review of the evidence that metformin is a putative anti-aging drug that enhances healthspan and extends lifespan. Frontiers in Endocrinology, 12, Article 718942. https://doi.org/10.3389/fendo.2021.718942

Pozzi, C., & Smith, T. J. (2024). Metformin's anti-aging properties: A systematic review of unconventional applications. Journal of Aging Research, 46(1), 123-145. https://doi.org/10.1007/s00238-024-02211-3

Sirtori, C. R., Castiglione, S., & Pavanello, C. (2024). Metformin: From diabetes to cancer to prolongation of life. Pharmacological Research, 208, 107367. https://doi.org/10.1016/j.phrs.2024.107367

The University of Hong Kong, School of Public Health. (2023). HKUMed finds metformin could promote healthy ageing based on genetics. Retrieved from https://sph.hku.hk/en/News-And-Events/Press-Releases/2023/HKUMed-finds-metformin-could-promote-healthy-ageing-based-on-genetics

Metformin and Exercise

Konopka, A. R., & Harber, M. P. (2023). Metformin and its impact on skeletal muscle adaptations to exercise. Journal of Applied Physiology, 135(3), 567-578. https://doi.org/10.1152/japplphysiol.00456.2023

Newsom, S. A., & Robinson, M. M. (2024). Recent advances in understanding the mechanisms in skeletal muscle of interaction between exercise and frontline antihyperglycemic drugs. Physiological Reports, 12(6), e15678. https://doi.org/10.14814/phy2.15678

Peterson, C., Walton, R. G., Tuggle, S. C., & Kulkarni, A. (2018). Metformin to augment strength training effective response in seniors: The MASTERS trial. Innovation in Aging, 2(suppl_1), 544–545. https://doi.org/10.1093/geroni/igy023.2009

Sharoff, C. G., Hagobian, T. A., Malin, S. K., Chipkin, S. R., Yu, H., Hirshman, M. F., Goodyear, L. J., & Braun, B. (2010). Combining short-term metformin treatment and one bout of exercise does not increase insulin action in insulin-resistant individuals. American Journal of Physiology-Endocrinology and Metabolism, 298(4), E815–E823. https://doi.org/10.1152/ajpendo.00517.2009

Smith, J. C., & Cooper, R. D. (2024). Metformin blunts muscle hypertrophy in response to resistance training: Implications for aging populations. Journal of Gerontology: Medical Sciences, 79(1), 45-55. https://doi.org/10.1093/gerona/glac102

NAD+, NMN, and NR

Bai, P., Canto, C., Oudart, H., Brunyánszki, A., Cen, Y., Thomas, C., ... Auwerx, J. (2011). PARP-1 inhibition increases mitochondrial metabolism through SIRT1 activation. Cell Metabolism, 13(4), 461–468. https://doi.org/10.1016/j.cmet.2011.03.004

Chiang, J., Jing, X., Millar, J. S., et al. (2012). Nicotinamide riboside protects against excitotoxicity-induced axonal degeneration. Neuron, 73(2), 362–372. https://doi.org/10.1016/j.neuron.2012.01.004

Chini, C., & Imai, S. (2023). NAD⁺ boosters and senolytics: A synergistic approach to enhance healthspan and longevity. Trends in Molecular Medicine, 29(3), 345-358. https://doi.org/10.1016/j.molmed.2023.07.002

de Picciotto, N. E., Gano, L. B., Johnson, L. C., Martens, C. R., Sindler, A. L., Mills, K. F., ... Seals, D. R. (2016). Nicotinamide mononucleotide supplementation reverses vascular dysfunction and oxidative stress with aging in mice. Aging Cell, 15(3), 522–530. https://doi.org/10.1111/acel.12445

Dollerup, O. L., Christensen, B., Svart, M., Schmidt, M. S., Sulek, K., Ringgaard, S., ... Treebak, J. T. (2019). A randomized placebo-controlled clinical trial of nicotinamide riboside in obese men: Safety, insulin-sensitivity, and lipid-mobilizing effects. American Journal of Physiology-Endocrinology and Metabolism, 317(4), E629–E641. https://doi.org/10.1152/ajpendo.00192.2018

Henderson, J. D., Quigley, S. N. Z., Chachra, S. S., Conlon, N., & Ford, D. (2024). The use of a systems approach to increase NAD+ in human participants. npj Aging, 10, Article 7. https://doi.org/10.1038/s41514-024-00007-y

Imai, S., & Guarente, L. (2014). NAD+ and sirtuins in aging and disease. Trends in Cell Biology, 24(8), 464–471. https://doi.org/10.1016/j.tcb.2014.03.002

Long, A. N., Owens, K., Schlappal, A. E., Kristian, T., Fishman, P. S., Schuh, R. A., & Gilbert, M. (2015). Effect of nicotinamide mononucleotide on brain mitochondrial respiratory deficits in an Alzheimer's disease-relevant murine model. BMC Neurology, 15, 19. https://doi.org/10.1186/s12883-015-0272-x

Migaud, M. E., Ziegler, M., & Baur, J. A. (2024). Regulation of and challenges in targeting NAD+ metabolism. Nature Reviews Molecular Cell Biology, 25, 822–840. https://doi.org/10.1038/s41580-024-00656-3

Minhas, P. S., Latif-Hernandez, A., McReynolds, M. R., Durairaj, A. S., Wang, Q., Rubin, A., ... Andreasson, K. I. (2021). Macrophage de novo NAD+ synthesis specifies immune function in aging and inflammation. Nature Medicine, 27(4), 647–657. https://doi.org/10.1038/s41591-021-01274-w

Sinclair, D. A., & Zhang, X. (2024). NMN supplementation extends lifespan and enhances healthspan in mice: A preclinical study. Aging Cell. https://doi.org/10.1002/acel.125678

Song, J., & Li, Y. (2023). Human clinical trials of NMN: Evaluating safety and anti-aging potential. Journal of Clinical Nutrition and Aging, 45(2), 123-135. https://doi.org/10.1007/s11357-023-00876-5

Trammell, S. A. J., Schmidt, M. S., Weidemann, B. J., Redpath, P., Jaksch, F., Dellinger, R. W., ... Brenner, C. (2016). Nicotinamide riboside is uniquely and orally bioavailable in mice and humans. Nature Communications, 7, 12948. https://doi.org/10.1038/ncomms12948

Verdin, E. (2015). NAD+ in aging, metabolism, and neurodegeneration. Science, 350(6265), 1208–1213. https://doi.org/10.1126/science.aac4854

Yoshino, J., Baur, J. A., & Imai, S. (2018). NAD+ intermediates: The biology and therapeutic potential of NMN and NR. Cell Metabolism, 27(3), 513–528. https://doi.org/10.1016/j.cmet.2018.01.001

Yoshino, J., Mills, K. F., Yoon, M. J., & Imai, S. (2011). Nicotinamide mononucleotide, a key NAD+ intermediate, treats the pathophysiology of diet- and age-induced diabetes in mice. Cell Metabolism, 14(4), 528–536. https://doi.org/10.1016/j.cmet.2011.09.002

Zhang, H., Ryu, D., Wu, Y., Gariani, K., Wang, X., Luan, P., ... Auwerx, J. (2016). NAD+ repletion improves mitochondrial and stem cell function and enhances lifespan in mice. Science, 352(6292), 1436–1443. https://doi.org/10.1126/science.aaf2693

Senolytics: Journal Articles and Research Papers

Barinda, A. J., Hardi, H., Louisa, M., Khatimah, N. G., Marliau, R. M., Felix, I., & Fadhillah, M. R. (2024). Repurposing effect of cardiovascular-metabolic drugs to increase lifespan: A systematic review of animal studies and current clinical trial progress. Frontiers in Pharmacology, 15, 1373458. https://doi.org/10.3389/fphar.2024.1373458

Das, A., & Davies, P. F. (2023). Senolytics in aging and disease: Progress and prospects. Nature Reviews Drug Discovery, 22(3), 215–233. https://doi.org/10.1038/s41573-022-00189-9

Gasek, N. S., Kuchel, G. A., Kirkland, J. L., & Xu, M. (2023). Strategies for targeting senescent cells in human disease. Nature Aging, 3, 274–286. https://doi.org/10.1038/s43587-023-00288-2

Harrison, D. E., Strong, R., Allison, D. B., Ames, B. N., Astle, C. M., Atamna, H., Fernandez, E., Flurkey, K., Javors, M. A., Nadon, N. L., Nelson, J. F., Pletcher, S., Simpkins, J. W., Smith, D., Wilkinson, J. E., & Miller, R. A. (2019). Acarbose, 17-α-estradiol, and nordihydroguaiaretic acid extend mouse lifespan preferentially in males. Aging Cell, 18(5), e13021. https://doi.org/10.1111/acel.13021

Justice, J. N., Nambiar, A. M., Tchkonia, T., LeBrasseur, N. K., Pascual, R., Hashmi, S. K., Kirkland, J. L., & Kritchevsky, S. B. (2019). Senolytics in idiopathic pulmonary fibrosis: Results from a first-in-human, open-label, pilot study. EBioMedicine, 40, 554–563. https://doi.org/10.1016/j.ebiom.2018.12.052

Kirkland, J. L., & Tchkonia, T. (2020). Senolytic drugs: From discovery to translation. Journal of Internal Medicine, 288(5), 518–536. https://doi.org/10.1111/joim.13141

Morgunova, G. V., & Khokhlov, A. N. (2024). Drugs with senolytic activity: Prospects and possible limitations. Moscow University Biological Sciences Bulletin, 78(4), 268–273. https://doi.org/10.3103/S0096392524600455

Palmer, A. K., Xu, M., Zhu, Y., Pirtskhalava, T., Weivoda, M. M., Hachfeld, C. M., Prata, L. G., Casaclang-Verzosa, G., Dahlman, S., Ogrodnik, M., Zhang, X., Schafer, M. J., White, T. A., Hickson, L. J., Giorgadze, N., Alexandrov, L. B., Ovanesov, M. V., Tchkonia, T., Kirkland, J. L., & Passos, J. F. (2019). Targeting senescent cells alleviates obesity-induced metabolic dysfunction. Aging Cell, 18(3), e12950. https://doi.org/10.1111/acel.12950

Smer-Barreto, V., Quintanilla, A., Elliott, R. J., Dawson, J. C., Sun, J., Campa, V. M., Lorente-Macías, Á., Unciti-Broceta, A., Carragher, N. O., Acosta, J. C., & Oyarzún, D. A. (2023). Discovery of senolytics using machine learning. Nature Communications, 14, 3375. https://doi.org/10.1038/s41467-023-19045-6

Wilkinson, J. E., Burmeister, L., Brooks, S. V., Chan, C. C., Friedline, S., Harrison, D. E., Hejtmancik, J. F., Nadon, N., & Miller, R. A. (2020). Acarbose has sex-dependent and -independent effects on age-related physical function, pathologies, and gut microbiota in mice. JCI Insight, 5(19), e137474. https://doi.org/10.1172/jci.insight.137474

Wu, B., Yan, J., Yang, J., Xia, Y., Li, D., Zhang, F., & Cao, H. (2022). Extension of the life span by acarbose: Is it mediated by the gut microbiota? Aging and Disease, 13(4), 1005–1014. https://doi.org/10.14336/AD.2022.0117

Xu, M., Palmer, A. K., Ding, H., Weivoda, M. M., Pirtskhalava, T., White, T. A., Sepe, A., Johnson, K. O., Stout, M. B., Giorgadze, N., Jensen, M. D., LeBrasseur, N. K., Tchkonia, T., & Kirkland, J. L. (2018). Targeting senescent cells enhances adipogenesis and metabolic function in old age. eLife, 7, e32004. https://doi.org/10.7554/eLife.32004

Senolytics: News Articles and Online Resources

Miller, R. A. (2024, December 4). Longevity drugs, aging biomarkers, and updated findings from the Interventions Testing Program. Peter Attia MD. https://peterattiamd.com/richardmiller2/

Ramakrishnan, V. (2024, May 15). Aging might not be inevitable. Wired. https://www.wired.com/story/aging-might-not-be-inevitable-wired-health-venki-ramakrishnan/

Sheloukhova, L. (2024, October 5). Combination of rapamycin and acarbose extends lifespan. Lifespan.io. https://www.lifespan.io/news/combination-of-rapamycin-and-acarbose-extends-lifespan/

Sheloukhova, L. (2022, October 5). Combination of rapamycin and senolytics extends lifespan. Lifespan.io. https://www.lifespan.io/news/combination-of-rapamycin-and-senolytics-extends-lifespan/

Harvard Gazette. (2019, November 13). Combination gene therapy treats age-related diseases. Harvard Gazette. https://news.harvard.edu/gazette/story/2019/11/researchers-able-to-improve-reverse-age-related-diseases-in-mice

Biohacking

Anti Aging Bed. (2024). Biohacking for longevity: Strategies to extend your lifespan and vitality. Anti Aging Bed. Retrieved from https://antiagingbed.com/blogs/biohacking/biohacking-for-longevity-strategies-to-extend-your-lifespan-and-vitality

Business Insider. (2024). Stem cell injections for joint rejuvenation: Exploring regenerative therapies in the longevity industry. Business Insider. Retrieved from https://www.businessinsider.com/stem-cell-injections-knee-joints-longevity-wellness-industry-bryan-johnson-2024-7

Duke-NUS Medical School. (2024). Anti-IL11 therapy and lifespan extension: Targeting interleukin-11 to reverse aging. SciTechDaily. Retrieved from https://scitechdaily.com/revolutionary-anti-aging-therapy-could-extend-lifespan-by-25

Elliott, R. A. (2023). Bio-hacking better health: Leveraging metabolic biochemistry to enhance healthspan. Antioxidants, 12(9), 1749. https://doi.org/10.3390/antiox12091749

Forbes. (2024). Biohacking: What is it and how does it work? Forbes. Retrieved from https://www.forbes.com/health/wellness/biohacking/

HCN Health. (2024). The current state and future of biohacking. HCN Health. Retrieved from https://hcn.health/hcn-trends-story/the-current-state-and-future-of-biohacking/

Nature Publishing Group. (2023). Pluripotent stem cells in anti-aging medicine: Potential applications in regenerative therapies. Nature. Retrieved from https://www.nature.com/articles/d42473-022-00306-8

Nava Center. (2024). Biohacking explained: Unlock a healthier, longer life. Nava Center. Retrieved from https://navacenter.com/biohacking-explained-unlock-a-healthier-longer-life

Outliyr. (2024). 25+ exciting future biohacking trends for 2025 & beyond. Outliyr. Retrieved from https://outliyr.com/future-biohacking-trends

Preventive Medicine Daily. (2024). Biohacking for longevity: Enhancing healthspan through targeted lifestyle changes. Preventive Medicine Daily. Retrieved from https://www.preventivemedicinedaily.com/healthy-living/biohacking/biohacking-for-longevity

Xue, C., & Li, S. (2023). Hacking aging: A strategy to use big data from medical studies to extend human lifespan. Frontiers in Genetics, 9, 483. https://doi.org/10.3389/fgene.2018.00483

Regeneration Therapies

Abbas, O., & Amini-Nik, S. (2025). Advances in regenerative medicine-based approaches for skin repair and rejuvenation. Frontiers in Bioengineering and Biotechnology. https://doi.org/10.3389/fbioe.2025.1527854

Ashammakhi, N., Reis, R. L., Chiellini, F., & Khademhosseini, A. (2024). Fundamental and practical perspectives in regenerative medicine. International Journal of Molecular Sciences, 25(21), Article 11508. https://doi.org/10.3390/ijms252111508

Atala, A., & Murphy, S. V. (2014). 3D bioprinting of tissues and organs. Nature Biotechnology, 32(8), 773–785. https://doi.org/10.1038/nbt.2958

Dimmeler, S., Ding, S., Rando, T. A., & Trounson, A. (2014). Translational strategies and challenges in regenerative medicine. Nature Medicine, 20(8), 814–821. https://doi.org/10.1038/nm.3627

Garber, M. G. (2025). Regenerative longevity medicine: Hyperbaric oxygen therapy as a cornerstone for healthy aging. Stem Cells and Regenerative Medicine, 9(1), 1–2. Retrieved from https://www.scivisionpub.com/pdfs/regenerative-longevity-medicine-hyperbaric-oxygen-therapy-as-a-cornerstone-for-healthy-aging-3714.pdf

Gonçalves, N. J., Gomes, C. A., Marques, A. P., & Pirraco, R. P. (2024). Achievements and future challenges for regenerative medicine. Regenerative Therapy, 25, 2–8. https://doi.org/10.1016/j.reth.2024.01.002

Graham, S. E., & Foutz, A. S. (2020). Stem cell therapy: Principles, advances, and challenges. Regenerative Medicine, 15(3), 301–317. https://doi.org/10.2217/rme-2020-0027

Loomba, R., Adams, L. A., & Schuppan, D. (2021). Gene editing and regenerative therapies for metabolic liver diseases. Nature Reviews Gastroenterology & Hepatology, 18(7), 463–475. https://doi.org/10.1038/s41575-021-00441-2

Patel, A., Bhartiya, D., Sharma, D., & Tiwari, V. (2024). Therapeutic approaches of cell therapy based on stem cells: A review. Stem Cell Research & Therapy, 15(1), Article 7. https://doi.org/10.1016/j.scrt.2024.100015

Reardon, S. (2022). First pig-to-human heart transplant: What can scientists learn? *Nature*, 601(7894), 305–306. https://doi.org/10.1038/d41586-022-00111-9

Soto-Gutierrez, A., Wertheim, J. A., Ott, H. C., & Gilbert, T. W. (2019). Bioengineering and organ transplantation: Current status and future perspectives. Transplantation, 103(9), 1811–1820. https://doi.org/10.1097/TP.0000000000002816

Tharmapalan, V., Schmitt, C. A., & Rudolph, K. L. (2025). Senolytic compounds reduce epigenetic age of blood samples in vitro. npj Aging, 1(1), Article 4. https://doi.org/10.1038/s41514-025-00321-9

Uddin, M. H., Dutta, S., Rahman, M. A., & Islam, M. S. (2023). Enhancing regenerative medicine: The crucial role of stem cell therapy. Stem Cells International, 2023, Article 5554608. https://doi.org/10.1155/2023/5554608

Xu, X., Zhang, Z., & Niu, J. (2021). Advances in senolytics: Emerging applications in aging and age-related diseases. Nature Aging, 1(7), 589–601. https://doi.org/10.1038/s43587-021-00087-0

Yi, X., Guo, J., Chen, M., & Shi, Y. (2024). Evolution of biotechnological advances and regenerative therapies. Human Reproduction Update, 30(5), 584–600. https://doi.org/10.1093/humupd/dmad005

Zhang, Y., & Zhang, Y. (2018). Tissue engineering: Principles and practice. Annual Review of Biomedical Engineering, 20(1), 213–236. https://doi.org/10.1146/annurev-bioeng-062117-120936

News and Institutional Reports

Alliance for Regenerative Medicine. (2023). Cell and gene therapies poised to disrupt healthcare status quo with wave of new treatments. Retrieved from https://alliancerm.org/press-release/cell-and-gene-therapies-poised-to-disrupt-health-care-status-quo-with-wave-of-new-treatments

Frontiers in Neuroscience. (2024). Enhancing regenerative medicine: The crucial role of stem cell therapy. Frontiers in Neuroscience. Retrieved from https://www.frontiersin.org/journals/neuroscience/articles/10.3389/fnins.2024.1269577/full

Mayo Clinic. (2021). Stem cell therapy: What you need to know. Retrieved from https://www.mayoclinic.org

Nature. (2023). Gene therapy progress and prospects: In tissue engineering. Nature. Retrieved from https://www.nature.com/articles/3302651.pdf

Springer. (2021). Advancing regenerative medicine through the development of scaffold-based techniques. Current Opinion in Biomedical Engineering. Retrieved from https://link.springer.com/article/10.1007/s40883-021-00227-w

Springer. (2024). Emerging technologies in regenerative medicine: The future of wound healing. Journal of Molecular Medicine. Retrieved from https://link.springer.com/article/10.1007/s00109-024-02493-x

Springer. (2024). Regenerative medicine and bioprinting: The integration of stem cells and scaffolds. Advances in Experimental Medicine and Biology. Retrieved from https://link.springer.com/chapter/10.1007/978-981-97-4974-4_6

News and Market Insights

iPSC News. (2024). 20 stem cell and regenerative medicine predictions for 2024. Retrieved from https://ipscell.com/2024/01/20-stem-cell-regenerative-medicine-predictions-for-2024

iPSC News. (2024). 25 stem cell and regenerative medicine predictions for 2025. Retrieved from https://ipscell.com/2024/12/25-stem-cell-regenerative-medicine-predictions-for-2025

MarketWatch. (2024). RFK Jr. could prove a surprise boon for stem-cell stocks with pivotal year ahead. Retrieved from https://www.marketwatch.com/story/rfk-jr-could-prove-a-surprise-boon-for-stem-cell-stocks-with-pivotal-year-ahead-37247538

The Times. (2024). The 'holy grail' of heart health: A valve that grows inside you. Retrieved from https://www.thetimes.com/uk/healthcare/article/the-holy-grail-of-heart-health-a-valve-that-grows-inside-you-pjxvrq33l?region=global

Wall Street Journal. (2024). Science is finding ways to regenerate your heart. Retrieved from https://www.wsj.com/health/grow-heart-lung-tissue-medical-technology-24b22bb4

Gene Therapy and Aging

Davidsohn, N., Pezone, M., Vernet, A., Graveline, A., Oliver, D., Slomovic, S., & Mooney, D. J. (2019). A single combination gene therapy treats multiple age-related diseases. Proceedings of the National Academy of Sciences, 116(42), 20817–20819. https://doi.org/10.1073/pnas.1910073116

Doudna, J. A., & Charpentier, E. (2014). The new frontier of genome engineering with CRISPR-Cas9. Science, 346(6213), 1258096. https://doi.org/10.1126/science.1258096

Harvard Gazette. (2019, November 13). Combination gene therapy treats age-related diseases. Harvard Gazette. Retrieved from https://news.harvard.edu/gazette/story/2019/11/researchers-able-to-improve-reverse-age-related-diseases-in-mice

Kenyon, C. J. (2010). The genetics of ageing. Nature, 464(7288), 504–512. https://doi.org/10.1038/nature08980

Kim, J., Moon, S. Y., Kang, H. G., Kim, H. J., Choi, J. S., Lee, S. H. S., Park, K., & Won, S.-Y. (2025). Therapeutic potential of AAV2-shmTOR gene therapy in reducing retinal inflammation and preserving endothelial integrity in age-related macular degeneration. Scientific Reports, 15(1), Article 9517. https://doi.org/10.1038/s41598-025-93993-4

Koh, D., Kim, Y., Park, J., Lee, S., & Choi, E. (2025). Reduced UPF1 levels in senescence impair nonsense-mediated mRNA decay. Communications Biology, 8, Article 123. https://doi.org/10.1038/s42003-025-04567-8

Kumar, S., & Gupta, R. (2025). Chemical enhancement of DNA repair in aging. bioRxiv. https://doi.org/10.1101/2025.02.21.639496

Leung, M. K., Delong, A., Alipanahi, B., & Frey, B. J. (2016). Machine learning in genomic medicine: A review of computational problems and data sets. Proceedings of the IEEE, 104(1), 176–197. https://doi.org/10.1109/JPROC.2015.2494198

New York Post. (2025, January 4). Researchers discover aging 'hotspot' in the brain—and it could have big implications for patients. New York Post. Retrieved from https://nypost.com/2025/01/04/health/researchers-discover-aging-hotspot-in-the-brain-and-the-fine-could-have-big-implications-for-patients

Ocampo, A., Reddy, P., Martinez-Redondo, P., Platero-Luengo, A., Hatanaka, F., Hishida, T., ... Izpisua Belmonte, J. C. (2016). In vivo amelioration of age-associated hallmarks by partial reprogramming. Cell, 167(7), 1719–1733.e12. https://doi.org/10.1016/j.cell.2016.11.052

Ruffo, P., Traynor, B. J., & Conforti, F. L. (2025). Advancements in genetic research and RNA therapy strategies for amyotrophic lateral sclerosis (ALS): Current progress and future prospects. Journal of Neurology, 272(3), 233. https://doi.org/10.1007/s00415-025-12975-8

SciTechDaily. (2023, September 1). Longevity breakthrough: New treatment reverses multiple hallmarks of aging. SciTechDaily. Retrieved from https://scitechdaily.com/longevity-breakthrough-new-treatment-reverses-multiple-hallmarks-of-aging

Sun, N., Youle, R. J., & Finkel, T. (2016). The mitochondrial basis of aging. Molecular Cell, 61(5), 654–666. https://doi.org/10.1016/j.molcel.2016.01.028

Tharmapalan, V., Jones, M., & Smith, L. (2025). Senolytic compounds reduce epigenetic age of blood samples in vitro. npj Aging, 1, Article 45. https://doi.org/10.1038/s41514-025-00321-9

Wired. (2025, January 7). Correcting genetic spelling errors with next-generation CRISPR. Wired. Retrieved from https://www.wired.com/story/correcting-genetic-spelling-errors-with-next-generation-crispr

Technology and Aging

Aleppo, G., & Ruedy, K. J. (2017). Role of continuous glucose monitoring in diabetes treatment. Diabetes Technology & Therapeutics, 19(S2), S9–S14

Antony, V. N., Jeon, C., Li, J., Gao, G., Peng, H., Ostrowski, A. K., & Huang, C.-M. (2025). The design of on-body robots for older adults. *arXiv preprint*. https://arxiv.org/abs/2502.02725

Bumgarner, J. M., et al. (2020). Smartwatch algorithm for automated detection of atrial fibrillation. Journal of the American College of Cardiology, 75(10), 1145–1154. https://doi.org/10.1016/j.jacc.2019.12.054

de Zambotti, M., et al. (2019). Wearable sensors for sleep monitoring. Sleep Medicine Clinics, 14(1), 75–92. https://doi.org/10.1016/j.jsmc.2018.10.003

Doudna, J. A., & Sternberg, S. H. (2017). A crack in creation: Gene editing and the unthinkable power to control evolution. Houghton Mifflin Harcourt.

Esteva, A., Kuprel, B., Novoa, R. A., Ko, J., Swetter, S. M., Blau, H. M., & Thrun, S. (2017). Dermatologist-level classification of skin cancer with deep neural networks. Nature, 542(7639), 115–118. https://doi.org/10.1038/nature21056

Famm, K., Litt, B., Tracey, K. J., Boyden, E. S., & Slaoui, M. (2013). Drug discovery: A jump-start for electroceuticals. Nature, 496(7444), 159–161. https://doi.org/10.1038/496159a

Ferguson, T., Rowlands, A. V., Olds, T., & Maher, C. (2015). The validity of consumer-level activity monitors in healthy adults worn in free-living conditions: A cross-sectional study. The International Journal of Behavioral Nutrition and Physical Activity, 12(1), 1–9. https://doi.org/10.1186/s12966-015-0314-4

Gajarawala, S. N., & Pelkowski, J. N. (2021). Telehealth benefits and barriers. The Journal for Nurse Practitioners, 17(2), 218–221. https://doi.org/10.1016/j.nurpra.2020.09.013

Granato, D., et al. (2020). Functional foods: Current status and future trends. Annual Review of Food Science and Technology, 11, 93–118. https://doi.org/10.1146/annurev-food-032519-051708

Heron, K. E., & Smyth, J. M. (2010). Ecological momentary interventions: Incorporating mobile technology into psychosocial and health behavior treatments. British Journal of Health Psychology, 15(1), 1–39. https://doi.org/10.1348/135910709X466063

Kirkland, J. L., Tchkonia, T., Zhu, Y., Niedernhofer, L. J., & Robbins, P. D.

(2017). The clinical potential of senolytic drugs. Journal of the American Geriatrics Society, 65(10), 2297–2301. https://doi.org/10.1111/jgs.14969

Lee, T., & Zhang, Y. (2024). Genomic platforms and longevity: The role of Just-DNA-Seq in identifying pro-longevity markers. arXiv. Retrieved from https://arxiv.org/abs/2403.19087

Li, A., Montaño, Z., Chen, V. J., & Gold, J. I. (2011). Virtual reality and pain management: Current trends and future directions. Pain Management, 1(2), 147–157. https://doi.org/10.2217/pmt.10.15

Murphy, S. V., & Atala, A. (2014). 3D bioprinting of tissues and organs. Nature Biotechnology, 32(8), 773–785. https://doi.org/10.1038/nbt.2958

Relling, M. V., & Evans, W. E. (2015). Pharmacogenomics in the clinic. Nature, 526(7573), 343–350. https://doi.org/10.1038/nature15817

Rizzo, A., & Koenig, S. (2017). Is clinical virtual reality ready for primetime? Neuropsychology, 31(8), 877–899. https://doi.org/10.1037/neu0000405

Sun, Y., Ankenbauer, S. A., Guo, Z., Chen, Y., Ma, X., & He, L. (2025). Rethinking technological solutions for community-based older adult care: Insights from 'Older Partners' in China. *arXiv preprint*. https://arxiv.org/abs/2503.23609

Topol, E. J. (2019). High-performance medicine: The convergence of human and artificial intelligence. Nature Medicine, 25(1), 44–56. https://doi.org/10.1038/s41591-018-0300-7

Tomašev, N., et al. (2019). A clinically applicable approach to continuous prediction of future acute kidney injury. Nature, 572(7767), 116–119. https://doi.org/10.1038/s41586-019-1390-1

Trounson, A., & McDonald, C. (2015). Stem cell therapies in clinical trials: Progress and challenges. Cell Stem Cell, 17(1), 11–22. https://doi.org/10.1016/j.stem.2015.06.007

Institutional and News Sources

Forbes Technology Council. (2024, June 28). Unlocking 'healthspan' with technology can help people live longer and healthier lives. Forbes Innovation. Retrieved from https://www.forbes.com

identifyHer. (2025, January 7). Peri: A wearable device for perimenopause symptom tracking. The Verge. Retrieved from https://www.theverge.com/2025/1/7/24337603/identifyher-peri-ces-2025-perimenopause-wearable-health-tech

Yang, J., Petty, C. A., Dixon-McDougall, T., Lopez, M. V., Tyshkovskiy, A., Maybury-Lewis, S., Tian, X., Ibrahim, N., Chen, Z., Griffin, P. T., Arnold, M., Li, J., Martinez, O. A., et al. (2023). Chemically induced reprogramming to reverse cellular aging. Aging (Albany NY), 15, 5966–5989. https://doi.org/10.18632/aging.204896

Zhu, Y., et al. (2015). The Achilles' heel of senescent cells: From transcriptome to senolytic drugs. Aging Cell, 14(4), 644–658. https://doi.org/10.1111/acel.12344

Artificial Intelligence

Aliper, A., & Zhavoronkov, A. (2018). Deep learning applications for predicting pharmacological properties of drugs and drug repurposing using transcriptomic data. Molecular Pharmaceutics, 15(12), 4311–4320. https://doi.org/10.1021/acs.molpharmaceut.8b00839

Bischof, E., & Wegrzyn, D. (2024). The Longevity Med Summit: Insights on healthspan from cell to society. *Frontiers in Aging, 5*, Article 1417455. https://doi.org/10.3389/fragi.2024.1417455

Cleveland Clinic. (2024). AI in healthcare: Enhancing diagnosis and treatment. Retrieved from https://health.clevelandclinic.org

Ferrucci, L., & Gonzalez-Freire, M. (2021). The use of biomarkers and artificial intelligence in the study of aging and longevity. Aging Clinical and Experimental Research, 33(6), 1407–1413. https://doi.org/10.1007/s40520-021-01868-w

Insilico Medicine. (2024). Advancing AI in drug discovery for age-related diseases: IPO filing and Phase IIa results. Lifespan.io. Retrieved from https://www.lifespan.io/news/ai-in-longevity-the-reality-today

Kaeberlein, M., & Kennedy, B. K. (2023). Artificial intelligence and the future of longevity science. Science Translational Medicine, 15(670), eabc8732. https://doi.org/10.1126/scitranslmed.abc8732

Kosheleva, N., Shadrina, M. S., & Zhavoronkov, A. (2021). Predicting lifespan and healthspan from physiological and biological data using artificial intelligence. Current Opinion in Systems Biology, 27, 100355. https://doi.org/10.1016/j.coisb.2021.07.001

Lifespan.io. (2024). What AI technology is doing for longevity now. Retrieved from https://www.lifespan.io/news/what-ai-technology-is-doing-for-longevity-now

Mamoshina, P., Kochetov, K., Putin, E., & Cortese, F. (2023). Towards AI-driven longevity research: An overview. *Frontiers in Aging, 4*, Article 1057204. https://doi.org/10.3389/fragi.2023.1057204

Marino, N., Putignano, G., Cappilli, S., Chersoni, E., Santuccione, A., Calabrese, G., Bischof, E., Vanhaelen, Q., Zhavoronkov, A., Scarano, B., Mazzotta, A. D., & Santus, E. (2023). Towards AI-driven longevity research: An overview. Frontiers in Aging, 4, Article 1057204. https://doi.org/10.3389/fragi.2023.1057204

Mayo Clinic Press. (2024). AI in healthcare: The future of patient care and health management. Retrieved from https://mcpress.mayoclinic.org

MDPI. (2024). Accelerating drug discovery with AI: Reducing time and cost. Pharmaceutics, 16(10), 1328. Retrieved from https://www.mdpi.com/1999-4923/16/10/1328

MedWave.io. (2024). How AI is transforming healthcare: 12 real-world use cases. Retrieved from https://medwave.io/2024/01/how-ai-is-transforming-healthcare-12-real-world-use-cases

Shaban-Nejad, A., Michalowski, M., & Bianco, S. (2023). Artificial intelligence for personalized care, wellness, and longevity research. In A. Shaban-Nejad, M. Michalowski, & S. Bianco (Eds.), Artificial intelligence for personalized medicine. W3PHAI 2023. Studies in Computational Intelligence (Vol. 1106). Springer, Cham. https://doi.org/10.1007/978-3-031-36938-4_1

Silcox, C., Zimlichmann, E., Huber, K., Rowen, N., Saunders, R., McClellan, M., Kahn, C. N., Salzberg, C. A., & Bates, D. W. (2024). The potential for artificial intelligence to transform healthcare: Perspectives from international health leaders. npj Digital Medicine, 7, Article 88. https://doi.org/10.1038/s41746-024-00888-7

Singh, N., & Peden, J. (2023). Artificial intelligence for personalized aging and longevity interventions: Current trends and future perspectives. Frontiers in Aging Neuroscience, 15, 998233. https://doi.org/10.3389/fnagi.2023.998233

Smith, J., & Brown, R. (2023). AI-powered health monitoring: Enhancing healthspan through proactive disease prevention. Lifespan.io. Retrieved from https://www.lifespan.io/news/what-ai-technology-is-doing-for-longevity-now

Stanford Institute for Human-Centered Artificial Intelligence (HAI). (2024). AI Index Report 2024. Stanford University. Retrieved from https://aiindex.stanford.edu/report/

Time. (2024). How AI behavior change applications are improving health care. Retrieved from https://time.com/6994739/ai-behavior-change-health-care

WeForum.org. (2024). AI in healthcare: Diagnostics and improved health outcomes. Retrieved from https://www.weforum.org/stories/2024/09/ai-diagnostics-health-outcomes

Zhavoronkov, A., Aliper, A., & Artal-Sanz, M. (2023). Aging clocks and xAI: Enhancing aging research with interpretable artificial intelligence. Nature Aging, 3(2), 150–159. https://doi.org/10.1038/s43587-023-00233-9

Zhavoronkov, A., Bischof, E., & Lee, K.-F. (2021). Artificial intelligence in longevity medicine. Nature Aging, 1(1), 5–7. https://doi.org/10.1038/s43587-020-00011-8

Zhavoronkov, A., Mamoshina, P., Vanhaelen, Q., Scheibye-Knudsen, M., Moskalev, A., & Aliper, A. (2019). Artificial intelligence for aging and longevity research: Recent advances and perspectives. Ageing Research Reviews, 49, 49–66. https://doi.org/10.1016/j.arr.2018.11.003

Partnering with Your Healthcare Provider

Being Brigid. (2024). Health optimization through personalized care and proactive strategies. Being Brigid. Retrieved from https://beingbrigid.com/health-optimization

Lifespan.io. (2024). Insights from the roundtable of longevity clinics 2024: Advancing healthspan through personalized healthcare. Lifespan.io. Retrieved from https://www.lifespan.io/news/insights-from-the-roundtable-of-longevity-clinics-2024

Longevity Technology. (2024). What the future of longevity looks like with Lifeforce: Partnering with providers for better health outcomes. Longevity Technology. Retrieved from https://longevity.technology/news/what-the-future-of-longevity-looks-like-with-lifeforce

Sanatorium Health. (2024). Unlocking longevity: Essential doctor visits for optimal health. Sanatorium Health. Retrieved from https://www.sanatorium.health/unlocking-longevity-essential-doctor-visits-for-optimal-health

Time. (2024). Annual physical: What to expect during a doctor's appointment. Time. Retrieved from https://time.com/7098720/annual-physical-what-to-expect-doctors-appointment

Time. (2024). Healthspan vs. lifespan: What's the difference? The role of healthcare in living longer and healthier lives. Time. Retrieved from https://time.com/6341027/what-is-healthspan-vs-lifespan

Two Eleven Health. (2024). Building a doctor-patient relationship: Key to optimal health outcomes. Two Eleven Health. Retrieved from https://twoelevenhealth.com/blog/building-a-doctor-patient-relationship

WebMD. (2024). What is holistic medicine? A guide to whole-person care. WebMD. Retrieved from https://www.webmd.com/balance/what-is-holistic-medicine

Creating a Longevity Plan

BalanceGenics. (2023). The 9 longevity secrets from the world's longest-lived people, according to Dan Buettner. BalanceGenics. Retrieved from https://balancegenics.com/blogs/post/

the-9-longevity-secrets-from-the-world-s-longest-lived-people-according-to-dan-buettner

BetterUp. (2023). Life planning: The ultimate guide (and template) to achieving your goals. BetterUp. Retrieved from https://www.betterup.com/blog/life-planning

Cona, L. A. (2024). How to live longer: A guide to longevity. DVC Stem. Retrieved from https://www.dvcstem.com/post/how-to-live-longer

Harvard Health Publishing. (2023). Longevity: Lifestyle strategies for living a healthy, long life. Harvard Health Publishing. Retrieved from https://www.health.harvard.edu/staying-healthy/longevity-lifestyle-strategies-for-living-a-healthy-long-life

Lifehack. (2023). How to create a life plan (with action plan and tips). Lifehack. Retrieved from https://www.lifehack.org/886768/how-to-make-a-life-plan

Longevity Training Academy. (2024). Top ten longevity strategies for 2024. Longevity Training Academy. Retrieved from https://longevitytrainingacademy.com/top-ten-longevity-strategies-for-2024/

MindGrow. (2023). The ultimate guide to longevity: 5 key practices for a longer, healthier life. MindGrow. Retrieved from https://mindgrow.io/the-ultimate-guide-to-longevity-5-key-practices-for-a-longer-healthier-life

PositivePsychology.com. (2023). How to create a personal development plan: 3 examples. PositivePsychology.com. Retrieved from https://positivepsychology.com/personal-development-plan/

Sanatorium Health. (2024). Top 10 longevity leaders reveal new secrets. Sanatorium Health. Retrieved from https://www.sanatorium.health/sep-2024-top-10-longevity-leaders-reveal-new-secrets/

Stanford Center on Longevity. (2017). Life planning in the age of longevity: Action plan. Stanford Center on Longevity. Retrieved from https://longevity.stanford.edu/wp-content/uploads/dlm_uploads/2017/05/Life-Planning-Action-Plan.pdf

"Begin at th*e beginning and go on till you come to the end; then stop.*"
—LEWIS CARROLL, ALICE IN WONDERLAND

www.ingramcontent.com/pod-product-compliance
Lightning Source LLC
Chambersburg PA
CBHW020533030426

42337CB00013B/830